Healing Yourself

Seventh Revised Edition

Joy Gardner

```
Printing History
    1st edition, 1972      500 copies
    2nd edition, 1973      500 copies
    3rd edition, 1973      500 copies
    4th edition, 1974    1,000 copies
    5th edition, 1975   10,000 copies
    6th edition, 1976   50,000 copies
    7th edition, 1980   38,000 copies

Total Printed          100,500 copies
```

The Crossing Press, Trumansburg, New York 14886

The medical information and advice contained in this book are based upon the experience and research of the author. Persons using this book should consult an appropriate health care provider when questions of medical treatment and care arise. The author and publisher assume no responsibility and are not liable for adverse effects resulting from the use of any advice or information contained in this book.

* * *

    This book, and particularly the Seventh Edition would not have been possible without Shari Basom, Rebecca Holcombe and Irmi Mende (assistance with practical realities), Mark Kent, Christine McCullough and Pippa Pedley (calligraphy), Steve Swann and Warren Baumgarten (cartoons), Mimi Kamp (herb drawings), Jane Beuscher (medical illustrations, Dr. Jim Campbell (pregnancy section), Kathy Karjala (nutritional adviser, Gary Dillon (front cover), Steve Johnson (back cover), and Eliza Schmidkunz (inspiration).

    Special thanks goes to Elaine and John Gill and the staff at The Crossing Press for being willing to take on this little book in its homespun version, and for the support and appreciation they've shown for this book and the ones to come.

Copyright c Joy Gardner, 1982

Library of Congress Cataloging-in-Publication Data

Gardner, Joy.
   Healing yourself.

   Bibliography: p.
   Includes index.
   1. self-care, Health.   2. Herbs--Therapeutic use.
3. Vitamin therapy. I. Title.
RA776.95.G37   1986   613   86-19663
ISBN 0-89594-213-5 (pbk.)

Healing Yourself is a simple manual on the use of herbs, vitamins, and other home remedies. When used as instructed, these remedies should be harmless, and beneficial to your body. All the suggestions given in this book have been used repeatedly, with good results. The book itself grew out of my experiences as herbal and nutritional consultant at the Country Doctor Clinic in Seattle, and elsewhere. Occasionally, someone will have an adverse reaction to a particular herb (just as some people are allergic to certain foods). I have tried to give warnings about such reactions that have occurred in the past, and I appreciate letters from readers which enable me to do this, as well as to continue upgrading the quality of information in each successive edition. We are, admittedly, being our own guinea pigs, but there is some comfort in knowing that healing herbs have been part of the human experiment for thousands of years. However, pregnant women should be particularly cautious; please see precautions on page 42.

This book is not meant to be a substitute for a good doctor. If you're sick, consult a doctor you trust. You may prefer a Naturopathic or Homeopathic Doctor, since they use mostly natural substances for healing. Once you have a reliable diagnosis, then you may want to try the remedies given in this book. Many clinics in the United States, Canada, and England now carry Healing Yourself and urge their patients to become more self-reliant by using it.

I suggest stocking your home with herbs and vitamins—as described under Home Remedy Self-Help Kit on pages 59-63—so that you can have on hand, at a reasonable cost, the means of dealing with most common ailments. In this way you can prevent colds and other simple disorders when the first symptoms occur, instead of waiting until a doctor can see you, or until these problems develop into serious disorders.

May you be in good health and good spirit. May you use this book well. May you nourish the people.

Joy Gardner

table of contents

please see index in back of book

Introduction
Table of Contents 1

COLD SYMPTOMS
    Colds, Prevention 2-3
    Aches & Pains 4
    Headaches 5
    Congestion & Sinuses 6
    Coughs 7
    Belly Aches 8
        gas
        stomach pain & flu
        upset stomach after meals
    Nausea & Vomiting 9
    Sore Throat 10-11
    Fever 12

Teeth 13

Asthma 14-15

BABIES AND SMALL CHILDREN:
    Problems & Diet
        colic 16
        cradle cap
        diaper rash
        foreskin infection 17
        teething
        food for infants
        strong teeth and bones

Constipation 18

Diarrhea 19

Hemorrhoids 20

Pinworms 21

Hepatitis 22-24

Hair Care 25

SKIN PROBLEMS
    Boils, Bruises 26
    Eczema, Psoriasis 27
    Burns
    Staph 28
    Pubic Area, Itching 29
    Herpes 30-31

Providing Nourishment:
    Dietary Guidelines 32-33

Nervous Tension 34
        Insomnia

Bladder Infections 35

WOMEN
    Vaginal Infections 36-37
    Cramps 38
        menstrual & IUD

BIRTH CONTROL
    The Ovulation Method 39-40
    Astrological Birth Control 40
    The Diaphragm 41

PREGNANCY & CHILDBIRTH 42-52
    Post-Natal Care 51
    Nursing 52

VITAMINS & MINERALS
    Vitamin A 53
    Vitamin B Complex 54-55
    Vitamin C 56
    Vitamin D
    Vitamin E 57
    Iron
    Calcium 58
    Magnesium

Home Remedy Self-Help Kit 59-63
    Terminology 63

Recommended Books 64

Your Own Remedies 65

Index 66

Dandelion

colds, prevention

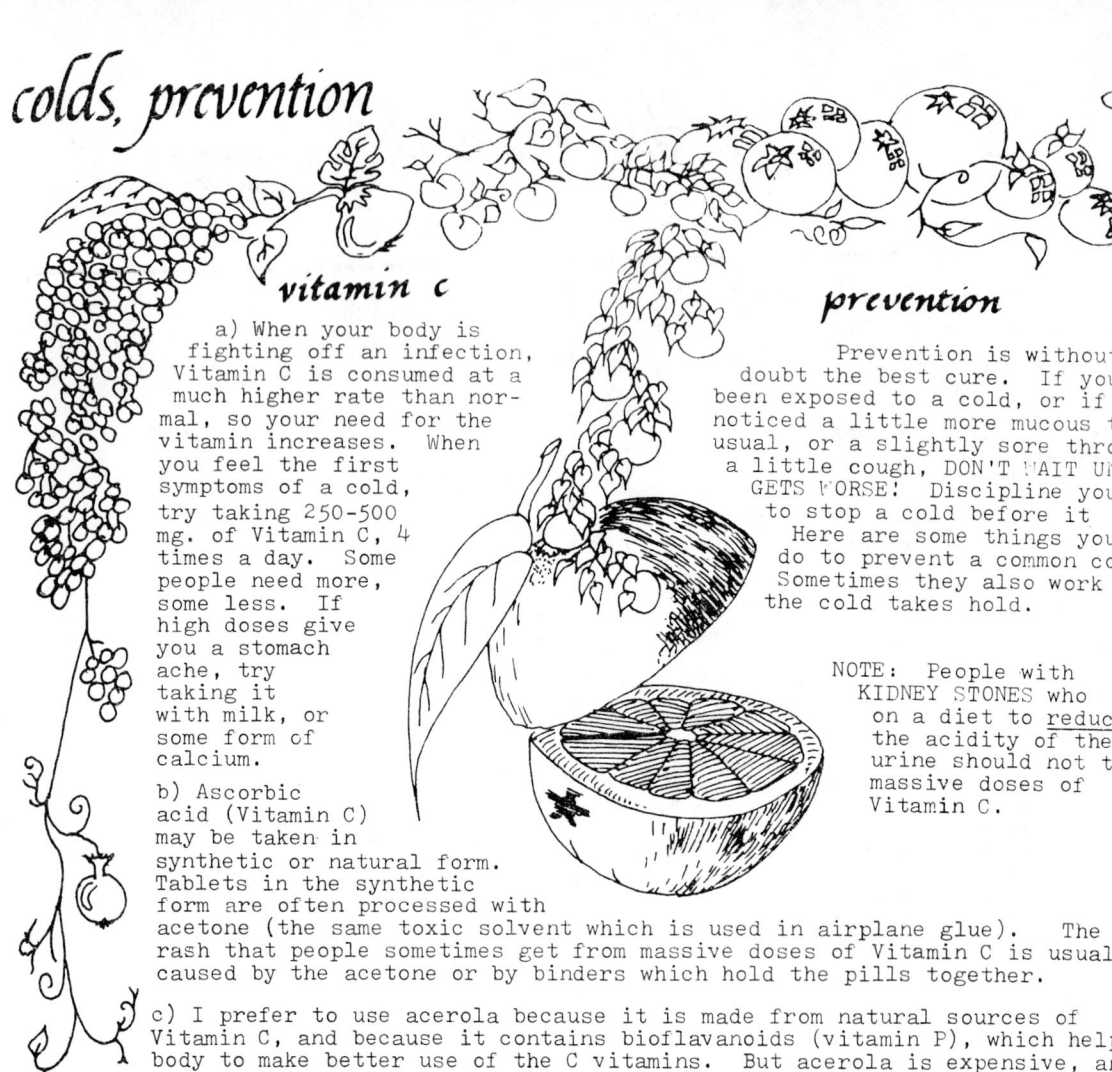

vitamin c

a) When your body is fighting off an infection, Vitamin C is consumed at a much higher rate than normal, so your need for the vitamin increases. When you feel the first symptoms of a cold, try taking 250-500 mg. of Vitamin C, 4 times a day. Some people need more, some less. If high doses give you a stomach ache, try taking it with milk, or some form of calcium.

b) Ascorbic acid (Vitamin C) may be taken in synthetic or natural form. Tablets in the synthetic form are often processed with acetone (the same toxic solvent which is used in airplane glue). The rash that people sometimes get from massive doses of Vitamin C is usually caused by the acetone or by binders which hold the pills together.

prevention

Prevention is without a doubt the best cure. If you've been exposed to a cold, or if you've noticed a little more mucous than usual, or a slightly sore throat, or a little cough, DON'T WAIT UNTIL IT GETS WORSE! Discipline yourself to stop a cold before it begins. Here are some things you can do to prevent a common cold. Sometimes they also work after the cold takes hold.

NOTE: People with KIDNEY STONES who are on a diet to reduce the acidity of their urine should not take massive doses of Vitamin C.

c) I prefer to use acerola because it is made from natural sources of Vitamin C, and because it contains bioflavanoids (vitamin P), which help the body to make better use of the C vitamins. But acerola is expensive, and so for massive doses, I suggest using ascorbic acid powder or granules (usually 1/4 tsp. contains 1000 mg. of Vitamin C, and it dissolves easily in water or juice). For bioflavanoids, take 1 acerola tablet, or eat green peppers or rose hips or the pulp and the white of organic oranges (the peels of sprayed oranges absorb huge amounts of dangerous pesticides).

d) When taking high doses of Vitamin C, reduce the dosage gradually, because high doses "teach" the kidneys to excrete the vitamin at a high level. So if you stop taking high doses suddenly, this may deplete the body of vitamin C. So if you've been taking 500 mg. 4 times a day, reduce to 250 mg. 4 times a day for 1-2 days, then 100 mg. 4 times a day, etc.

e) If you'd like to know whether you're getting enough vitamin C on any particular day, you can test your own urine. Since the body excretes any Vitamin C it doesn't need, the presence of Vitamin C in your urine indicates that you're getting enough. You can use VITAMIN C TEST PAPERS by moistening a small blue paper with a drop of urine. If it turns white, this indicates that there is Vitamin C in your urine. These papers are available from the Wholesale Nutrition Club, Box 1113, Sunnyvale, Calif. 94088. They also carry powdered vitamin C as Ascorbic Acid (an acid base), as Sodium Ascorbate (a salt base), and as Calicum Ascorbate (a calcium base). The Sodium Ascorbate is the least expensive.

colds, prevention *page two*

garlic

It's best to use organic garlic, since it's supposed to have more antibiotic properties.

    a) Chew a clove or two of garlic, 2 or 3 times a day, until the symptoms disappear -- and then for 2 or 3 more days. Or cut a clove into small pieces and swallow it down with water. Or spread it on your toast. Just be sure to eat a whole clove. It seems to be most effective when eaten raw (though brewing -- as with the tea -- doesn't seem to hurt it any).

    b) Garlic may also be taken by cutting a clove into tiny pieces and putting it into a 00 gelatin capsule (available in some drugstores and health food stores). It's best to do this just before taking the garlic, because the cut garlic is moist, and the capsule begins to dissolve when wet.

    c) GARLIC-AND-LEMON TEA is another solution if you don't savor the taste of raw garlic. This tea tastes good, even to children and most other people. Cut one small clove into tiny pieces and put in bottom of cup and squish with a spoon. Add juice of ¼ small lemon. Brew a cup of tea, preferably mint or peppermint for good taste (peppermint is a stronger healer). Put 1 tsp. tea per cup in the pot, add the garlic and lemon, and pour in the boiling water. Cover the pot and let brew for 3-5 minutes. Strain. Use honey as desired. Drink one cup, 3 times a day, until the symptoms disappear -- and then for 2 or 3 more days.

PARSLEY is a good antidote for the taste and smell of garlic.

hot apple cider vinegar & honey tea

    Add one cup boiling water to 2-3 Tbsp. apple cider vinegar and 2-3 Tbsp. honey. Drink as needed.

grandma's friendly advice

People with colds should try to avoid exposing others to their sickness.

    Don't share silverware, plates, cigarettes, etc.

Remember to turn your head away from other people when you cough or sneeze (germs die quickly in the air, but last a long time on your hands, so don't cover your mouth with your hand unless you're in a crowded place where you can't turn away).

Wash your hands frequently to avoid exposing others to your germs. Be especially careful after going to the bathroom, and before preparing food.

                            GET PLENTY OF REST

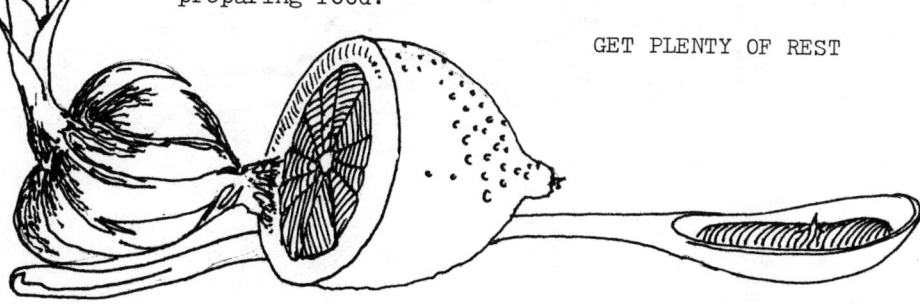

ACHES & PAINS

including:
- Aching muscles
- Strains
- Soreness
- Sprains
- Swellings
- Bumps
- Hits
- Bangs
- Falls

An excellent LINIMENT can be made, to deal with all of these things. Most people find that it brings relief in about 1/3 the time that such things would take to heal on their own. In many cases, it helps to rub it in for 15-20 minutes at a time, 3 or 4 times a day, to take out the soreness. If you can't rub directly over the spot, then rub around it until the soreness lessens. We've been told that it's also good to fight skin parasites - like scabies. It takes a week to make, so make some now so you'll have it when you need it. Here's the instructions (courtesy of Jethro Kloss, Back to Eden):

Ingredients: combine 1 oz. powdered myrrh, 1/2 oz. powdered golden seal, 1/4 oz. cayenne pepper, 1 pint rubbing alcohol (70%); mix together and let stand seven days, shake well every day, then pour liquid into another bottle (just the liquid, not the sediment), then cork.

Sometime an ache or a pain will be extremely intense in one small area. Another treatment, which stimulates circulation and breaks up congestion in small areas is TIGER BALM. It's oil of camphor in a petroleum base. It comes from China, and is available from the House of Rice in Seattle, and other places where Chinese items are sold. It costs about 35¢ for a small vial. Actually it's very similar to Ben Gay. You apply it to the area, and in about 10 minutes, you feel intense heat on that area. It's also excellent for breaking up congestions, when rubbed into the chest.

headaches

It's a good idea to avoid aspirin unless you really need it; it's a stronger drug than most people realize. But if you feel you have to have aspirin now and then, spend a little more money and buy Tylenol (<u>plain</u> acetomenophen -- products that mix this chemical with others, such as Excedrin, may be harmful). It's an aspirin substitute which has been proven to be much less harmful than aspirin, but usually just as effective for pain and fever -- but it's not useful for inflammation.

frontal headaches

Headaches in the front of the head almost always respond immediately to a firm massage at the back of the neck, at the base of the skull. The point (known in acupuncture as Gall Bladder 20, or Feng Chi) can be located at a level on the neck, just a little lower than the bottom of the ear lobes, and about midway between the ears and the spinal column, in a definite depression to the outside of the large vertical muscles at the back of the neck. Use the flat part of the thumb and middle finger, and keeping them in place, make a very firm, circular movement for up to 3 minutes (no longer, or you may reverse the effect).

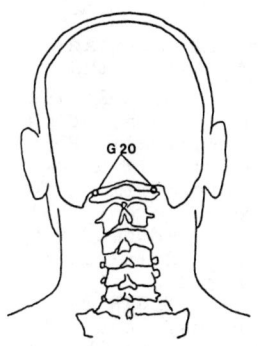

sinus headaches

Sinus headaches and those that accompany COLDS and CONGESTION respond well to TIGER BALM (a Chinese ointment -- camphor in a petroleum base -- a small vial costs about 35¢ and can usually be obtained from stores that sell Chinese products), rubbed into the temples and the area above the nose between the eyebrows (this is a sinus point known as Governing Vessel 24.5 or Yin Tang in acupuncture). After a few minutes, it creates a hot sensation and then you may begin to feel the congestion breaking up.

headaches ~ tightness of head, migraines

These can be treated effectively with the following time-honored remedy: rub peppermint oil (which can be purchased at a reasonable price at almost any drugstore) into the temples. If desired, it can be spread over the forehead, cheeks and neck. Relax. Lie down. Most people find that the tightness goes away quickly. Even MIGRAINES, in the beginning stage, often respond to peppermint oil. ESSENTIAL BALM contains peppermint oil and works very well for headaches. It comes in a small vial, costs 35¢, and can be purchased at some stores where Chinese items are sold.

The following TEAS are good for headaches, to ease the tension of nerves and muscles. Choose one, or combine them any way you like.

CATNIP, PEPPERMINT, or SAGE: cover 1 tsp. leaves with 1 cup
    boiling water and brew 5 minutes.

VALERIAN ROOT: cover 2 tsp. herb with 2 cups boiling water
    and brew 20 minutes. NOTE: Valerian Root is excellent
    for calming nerves, and is a fine sedative tea, but
    some people are allergic to it and get restless, nauseous,
    dizzy, or stomach aches from it. So just try a small
    amount the first time you use it.

See also page 34 on Nervous Tension.

Congestion & Sinuses:

People who are troubled with congestion should be particularly careful not to stay in overheated or over-air-conditioned rooms (68 degrees is a good temperature during the day), to get plenty of fresh air, and to sleep with the heat turned down or off. If radiators or wood or oil heaters are used, place a container of water on the heater, to keep moisture in the air and to keep the sinuses from getting dried out.

sinus congestion

Sinus congestion is often brought on by an allergy, so check out your house for feathers, dust, cats, and other things that could cause an allergic reaction. You may try to remove these things for a week, to see if the condition improves. Some good home treatments are:

1. EPHEDRA TEA (also known as desert tea, mormon tea, or squaw tea. Chinese Ephedra, or ma huang, is stronger, so substitute 3/4 tsp. for 1 tsp. in this recipe): Bring 2 cups of water to a boil, add ephedra, and simmer for 20 minutes. If using twigs, use a small handful. If using the granulated herb, use 2 tsps. Simmer for 20 minutes. Drink as needed. Warning: for small children, use only half as much (see note on page 14), and give ½ cup at a time.
2. FENUGREEK TEA: Use 1 tsp. per cup of boiling water -- simmer 20 minutes -- drink as needed. This herb is popular among naturopathic doctors for sinusitis.
3. TIGER BALM: This is a Chinese ointment made of camphor (and sometimes other herbs) in a petroleum base. It may be found in some health food stores, and places were Chinese items are sold. Apply to the area above the nose and between the eyes, to the temples, and wherever there is discomfort (see illustration of sinuses, below).

nasal congestion

Any one or all of the following may be used as decongestants, to clear the nasal passages and to enable you to breathe, which is especially helpful before going to bed:

1. EPHEDRA TEA: See above, under Sinus Congestion.
2. EUCALPTUS STEAM: Use 1 tsp. eucalyptus oil (available in most health food stores and drugstores) in a humidifier or vaporizer (see page 14), or use several eucalyptus leaves, a few 'nuts', and a small piece of the inner green bark from the tree (a handful of leaves will do, but it's not as potent). Simmer in 2 cups of water in a covered pot for 10 minutes. Then take the pot from the heat. Remove the lid, lean your head over the pot, cover your head and the pot with a towel, and inhale. You may have to come out from under the towel to exhale until it cools down a bit. Repeat until the steam is gone. Do this 2 or 3 times a day, as needed. The water may be saved and used again a couple of times. If using a humidifier or vaporizer, place it next to the bed in a closed room.

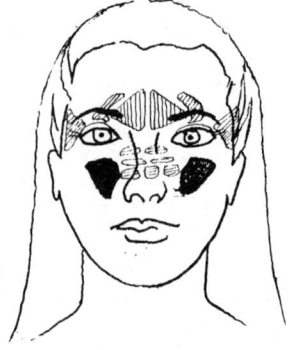

▨ FRONTAL
▤ ETHMOIDAL
▧ SPHENOIDAL
■ MAXILLARY

chest congestion

1. EPHEDRA TEA: See above, under Sinus Congestion.
2. TIGER BALM: See above, under Chest Congestion. Rub into the chest; you'll soon feel a sensation of warmth in your chest. Ben Gay can also be used the same way, to loosen up the phlegm. Tiger Balm comes in 2 types, red and white. The red is hotter, and more powerful, and works well on the chest. The white is milder, and usually preferred for the face.

coughs

1. COLTSFOOT COUGH SYRUP:
This syrup tastes real good; kids love it. Bring 1 cup of water to a boil. Add 3 Tbsp. coltsfoot leaves and simmer for 10 minutes. Strain and add $\frac{1}{4}$ cup honey (4 Tbsp.). Place on low heat until honey is dissolved. Then bottle and refrigerate. Add juice of $\frac{1}{4}$ lemon if desired. (If refrigeration is not available, use 1 cup of honey as a preservative.)

2. HOREHOUND COUGH SYRUP:
If your cough is really bad, this tastes strong and kind of bitter, but it's very effective to raise the phlegm and relieve the cough:

Boil 2 cups of water and add:
  1 Tbsp. comfrey root
Simmer 10 minutes and add:
    2 Tbsp. horehound
    1 Tbsp. mullein
    1 Tbsp. yerba santa
Simmer 10 more minutes -- remove from heat and add:
    1 Tbsp. peppermint
    1 Tbsp. chamomile or
       catnip
    1 Tbsp. yarrow
Brew 5 more minutes, then strain. Mix one part of this mixture with 2 parts honey (that's right) and stir until smooth. Add juice of $\frac{1}{2}$ lemon if desired. Drink freely, as needed. Refrigerate, or else leave it out and make a great beer. Either way, it's also excellent for sore throats and runny noses.

   If you still get that "ticklish" sensation in your throat, add some cayenne and brandy. Grampa will love it.

3. SAGE, GARLIC AND HONEY:
This tea is very effective for upper respiratory problems in general (colds, coughs, congestion of sinuses or lungs, sore throats), and as an expectorant (to help cough up phlegm), and to induce sweating.

Boil 6 cups of water and pour over:
    2 heaping Tbsp. sage leaves
    2 cloves garlic, chopped fine
      (preferably organic; more
      antibiotic properties)
    $\frac{1}{2}$ lemon (optional: throw in peel
      if it's organic -- lots of
      pesticides in the peel)
    plenty of honey
Steep for 5 minutes. For best results, fast and drink the tea hot, as much as 3 cups an hour. Then stay in bed with plenty of blankets and sweat.

4. CAYENNE:
This is excellent for a persistent, hacking cough. Fill 00 gelatin capsules (available in some drugstores or health food stores) with cayenne. Take one to two caps of cayenne, three times a day. (not recommended for people with stomach ulcers)

Belly-aches

gas... intestinal flu... pain in stomach, stomach flu, upset stomach after meals

gas

An excellent remedy for gas can be made by simmering 1 tsp. powdered or granulated slippery elm bark in 2 cups of water for 20 minutes. Strain and drink as needed. Sweeten as desired. Slippery elm also has a laxative effect. Note: this is an excellent remedy for pregnant women, contrary to rumors that claim that slippery elm is an abortive. In the old days, a piece of the whole bark was put up into the uterus as an irritant, to induce abortions. The tea, however, is very mild, being given to patients who can't hold anything else down on their stomach. In fact, it is said to be very healing to stomach ulcers (use as directed above).

stomach pain and flu

1. Combine equal parts of golden seal, slippery elm, cinnamon, and cayenne powders.* Put through a strainer to mix thoroughly. Fill 00 gelatin capsules (available in some drugstores and health food stores). Take one cap and follow with ½ glass of warm water (a cap holds ¼ tsp.) -- or put ¼ tsp. of the mixture on a butter knife and drop on the back of your tongue and swallow quick with warm water (it's bitter, but there aren't many tastebuds on the back of the tongue). Do this before each meal or as needed. Most people find it usually brings instant relief. It's a good thing to have already prepared and handy. One or two doses are usually enough, but it can be continued for a few days if necessary. (This remedy may not be desireable if there's vomiting, because the bitter taste of the golden seal keeps coming up. -- See also page 9 on Nausea & Vomiting.)

2. Hot apple cider vinegar and honey tea: Add one cup of boiling water to 2-3 Tbsp. apple cider vinegar and 2-3 Tbsp. honey. Drink as needed.

upset stomach after meals

If you have a chronic problem of upset stomach after meals, or a sickness that makes eating difficult --

1. Try one 00 cap of golden seal powder and one 00 cap of cayenne* with a whole cup of warm water, about ½ hour before each meal, to cleanse your stomach ... or

2. A few sips of gentian root infusion taken before meals will have a similar effect. Boil 2 cups of water, and add 3 tsps. gentian root, and simmer 20 minutes.

- - - - -

*Cayenne and Golden Seal are not recommended if you have stomach ulcers (see note above, under Gas, for Ulcers).

nausea

1. GENTIAN ROOT: You can chew on about ¼ tsp. (it's very bitter), or you can make a tea by adding 2 tsp. gentian root to 2 cups boiling water and simmering it for 20 minutes. Then you can add 1 tsp. peppermint, for flavor AND for nausea.

2. GOLDEN SEAL: ¼ tsp. in a 00 gelatin capsule (see remedy 1. on page 8 under Stomach Pain). Not advisable if nausea is accompanied by vomiting because the taste keeps coming up again. Safe for pregnant women, in this quantity, especially if the following advice is followed (which applies to everyone): always use Golden Seal with Vitamin C (to counteract toxicity) and follow with 2-3 Tbsp. yogurt or acidophilus (golden seal is said to destroy intestinal bacteria which manufacture Vitamin B -- these foods will restore such bacteria). ALSO GOOD FOR DIZZINESS.

3. PEPPERMINT TEA: Cover 1 tsp. tea with 1 cup boiling water. Brew for 5 minutes. ALSO GOOD FOR DIZZINESS.

vomiting

1. It often helps to swallow CRACKED ICE.

2. Some people find it desirable to fast and eat only YOGURT; <u>lots</u> of yogurt. Preferably plain yogurt. If you have to use a sweetner, use honey.

3. PEPPERMINT TEA: It settles the stomach and is nourishing. Cover 1 tsp. tea with 1 cup boiling water; brew for 5 minutes.

4. BARLEY WATER: A time-honored remedy which is bland, soothing, and nourishing. Place ½ cups barley in a strainer, rinse it well with cold water to remove any dust or impurities. Then add the barley to two cups of fresh water in a pot. Bring to a boil and simmer 10 minutes. Strain the water into a cup for the ill person, who should take it in small sips as tolerated. The cooked barley may be saved for use in soups etc.

5. SLIPPERY ELM TEA: This will often stay down on a stomach that can't hold anything else. Bring 2 cups of water to a boil, add 1 tsp. slippery elm bark (granulated or powdered), and simmer for 20 minutes. Strain if desired. Drink as needed. Also good for congestion and sore throats. For babies, use half as much. Slippery elm is also a mild laxative.

The easiest way to cure a sore throat is by stopping it in the first day or two. Don't put it off. Try the garlic or Vitamin C treatment described under COLDS, PREVENTION. But if you're too late

sore

throats

viral sore throats

These go away on their own, but here's how to relieve the symptoms and help speed recovery:

1. For an excellent THROAT LOZENGE, let a 500 mg. pill of ROSE HIPS or a 100 mg. tablet of ASCORBIC ACID (Vitamin C) dissolve in the back of your throat.

2. WARM SALT WATER GARGLES: add 1 tsp. salt to one quarter cup warm water. Gargle several times, and do this at least three times a day.

3. GOLDEN SEAL AND MYRRH: Combine four parts golden seal powder with 1 part myrrh powder. (Cayenne can be used instead of myrrh). Mix thoroughly. Fill 00 gelatin capsules (available in some drugstores or health food stores). Take 1 to 2 capsules, 3 times a day as needed. This is excellent for enlarged tonsils, mouth sores, and all kinds of throat troubles. Also take 100 mgs. Vitamin C, 3 times a day, to counteract any possibile toxicity from the golden seal, and follow with 2-3 Tbsp. yogurt or acidophilus: golden seal is said to destroy intestinal bacteria which manufacture Vitamin B. These foods will restore such bacteria. Note: wash the capsules down with ½ cup warm water or tea.

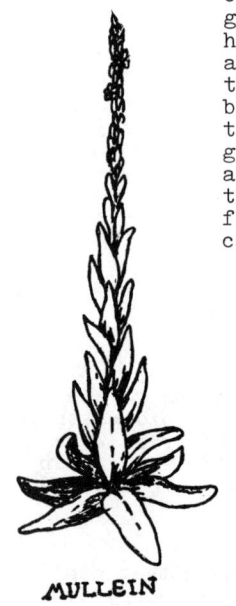
MULLEIN

4. GOOD TEAS: drink at least one cup every few hours and gargle with any one or combination of these teas:

COMFREY ROOT, BLACKBERRY ROOT, SLIPPERY ELM BARK, GINSENG ROOT: boil 2 cups of water and add 2 tsp. of any one or any combination of these herbs -- simmer 20 minutes. (With powdered herbs use half as much.)

MULLEIN TEA: boil 2 cups of water -- add 2 tsps. tea -- simmer 10 minutes

sore throats
page two

bacterial sore throats (strep ~ gonorrheal)

If you have a sore throat, and it doesn't get better in a day or two with one of the foregoing remedies, then see a doctor and have it cultured. If it's bacterial, it will probably have to be treated with antibiotics. When taking antibiotics, which are somewhat toxic, it's a good idea to take Vitamin C to counteract the toxicity: 100 mgs. 3 times a day. The antibiotics usually used to treat strep are non-specific, i.e., they kill some beneficial bacteria along with the strep, and may upset the natural balance of body bacteria, resulting in such deficiency diseases as yeast infections in women. After you've finished taking the antibiotics, then eat several Tablespoons of plain, unstabilized yogurt daily, for several days, to restore your normal intestinal bacteria. (Lactobacilli occur naturally in the vagina and intestines, and is the bacteria which is used to turn milk into yogurt.)

antibiotic alternatives

Rheumatic fever is a very serious disease which can develop as a complication of strep. This is one reason why antibiotics are always used by medical people for strep, and why patients are urged to continue taking antibiotics for about 10 days. Strep can be treated without antibiotics, but only if you're willing to exercise extreme caution. In 1934, Dr. Rinehart did some experiments that indicated that rheumatic fever occurred in the presence of strep only if there was also a deficiency of Vitamin C (<u>American Journal of Pathology</u>, 1934). His work was repeated by some members of the Public Health Service (<u>Public Health Reports</u>, March 16, 1934), but the experiments were limited, and therefore inconclusive. Unfortunately, this line of research was abandoned, probably because of the advent of antibiotics in the 1940's. Nevertheless, it seems advisable to take at least 500 mg. of Vitamin C per day for 10 days when treating strep. In addition to this, ALWAYS be sure to have a throat culture taken after the symptoms are gone, to be <u>sure</u> that the strep organism has been eliminated. If these precautions are observed, the following home treatments may be tried:

1. ALFALFA PILLS: This remedy almost always works to remove the symptoms of strep, within 24-48 hours. Adults take 10 pills and 100 mg. of Vitamin C every 3 hours, until symptoms are gone. Children 3-5 years old take 5 pills and 100 mg. of Vitamin C. Children 5-10 years old take 7-8 pills and 100 mg. of Vitamin C. I've found that Shaklee alfalfa pills are extremely effective, and are easy to swallow. They're available from Shaklee distributors, who can be found by looking in the yellow pages of a telephone directory, under Health Food Products or Cleaning Products (they sell both).

2. OIL OF BITTER ORANGE: Use a Q-Tip to apply the oil to the back of the throat. Cover thoroughly. Do this 3 times a day until all symptoms are gone, and then for another 2 days. This remedy is sometimes effective, but is less reliable than the alfalfa pills. Oil of Bitter Orange may be ordered from Nature's Herb Company, 281 Ellis Street, San Francisco, California 94102. or

3. "THOUSAND-YEAR-OLD EGGS" or PRESERVED DUCK EGGS: These are duck eggs which have been buried at least 6 months in bat dung, so that they are penetrated by spores which seem to be a natural source of penicillin. Yet people who are fatally allergic to penicillin have eaten these eggs without unpleasant side effects. However, one woman who was allergic to eggs did have a bad reaction. Peel the egg, then cut it up and cover with 1 Tbsp. soy sauce, 1 Tbsp. vegetable oil, and a pinch of powdered ginger. Divide 1 egg into 3 parts (4 parts for children; for infants, just divide the yolk into 3 parts), and eat 1 part at each meal. Adults usually use 3-4 eggs to clear up the symptoms of strep; children use 2-3. I recommend Four Seas Preserved Eggs, which are available in some Chinese grocery stores.

FEVER

Fever is considered present if the temperature is 100 degrees F. or more by mouth, or 101 degrees F. or more by rectum. Strenuous activity or emotional excitement or ovulation in women can cause a temporary rise in temperature. During a fever, a person should receive more than their normal intake of fluid, in order to reduce the possibility of dehydration (removal of water from the body, which can lead to shock or other severe side effects). If a fever stays above 102 degrees for adults, or 104 degrees for children, for over 24 hours, a doctor should be consulted. The situation is more likely to be dangerous in the case of an abrupt onset of fever (from normal to 103 degrees within an hour or two) which could indicate the presence of meningitis or some other serious illness, and a doctor should be contacted <u>immediately</u>.

If the need for aspirin is felt, we recommend Tylenol (plain acetomenophen) which is much less harmful than aspirin (acetylsalicylic acid). We suggest trying the following techniques first, since they do not interfere with the natural processes by which the body is already combatting the infection.

1. ALCOHOL RUBS: sponge the forehead, the temples, and -- if desired -- the whole body, with cotton soaked in alcohol every 15 minutes or half hour, until the fever goes down. In Harborview hospital, they place an ice bag on the forehead and a hot water bottle on the feet and then give an alcohol rub, going from the feet up to the heart.

2. COOL WATER: sponge off fevered person with cool (not cold) cloths. Or you can put a baby or an adult right in a tub or basin of cool water. You may want to begin with warm water, and then gradually add cold water to the basin or tub. When the person becomes chilled, take out of the tub, or take off the cloths, and hold the person wrapped in towels or cover with a blanket, but do not rub. Begin again when the chill passes. Do this in a warm (not hot) room with no drafts.

3. PEPPERMINT AND ELDER FLOWER TEA: Place 1/4 ounce peppermint leaves and 1/4 ounce elder flowers (or yarrow, but they're bitter) in a pottery or glass container. Boil 2 cups of water and pour over the herbs. Cover and steep for 15 minutes. Sweeten as desired -- strain -- drink warm -- go to bed. Usually the tension eases up and the fever goes away very quickly. Excellent for children, also. This tea works by opening the pores to let the toxins come out.

4. SAGE TEA: cover 1 tsp. sage tea with 1 cup of boiling water and brew for 5 minutes. Add honey as desired. Spearmint tea may be added to soften the flavor. Drink as needed.

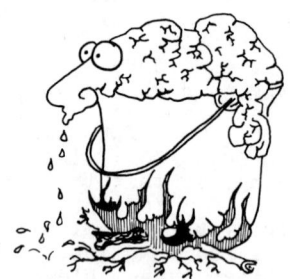

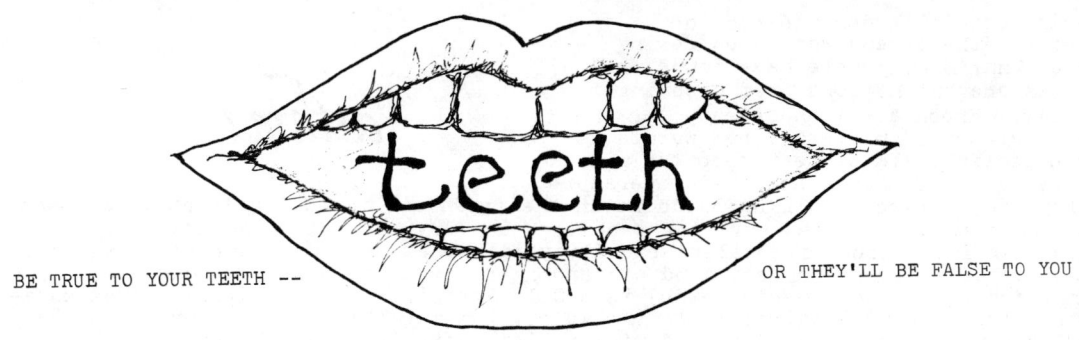

BE TRUE TO YOUR TEETH --   OR THEY'LL BE FALSE TO YOU

"What do you expect when 50 million bacteria go potty in your mouth every day?" -- anonymous dentist

toothache

If you have a toothache, get yourself to a dentist and have it fixed proper. But if you can't go right away, here are some good relief measures:

1. NIACIN: Take 50-100 mgs. of niacin. Some people get a niacin rush; flushing of the face, and a prickly sensation at the extremeties or all over the body. Don't panic; it will pass shortly. The niacin usually relieves the pain entirely. Niacin can also be taken as niacinamide with the rest of the B-Complex and will cause no reaction. Plus Products Formula 72 is a good source. It's also important to get plenty of Vitamin C, which by itself often relieves toothaches.

2. GARLIC: Place a piece of garlic in your mouth, behind the painful tooth, for an hour.

3. OIL OF CLOVES: This is a well-known local anaesthetic. The oil is a very concentrated form of cloves which is also irritant, so try not to get it on the gums. Soak a plug of cotton in the oil and then insert the cotton directly into the cavity.

gingivitis and pyorrhea and trenchmouth

These are different stages of gum degeneration, characterized by inflammation (redness and swelling) of the gums and sometimes bleeding (gingivitis), sometimes pus, with progressive cell death and loosening of the teeth (pyorrhea), even leading to sore throat and mouth, swelling of the lymph nodes in the neck, foul and offensive breath, painful swallowing (trenchmouth -- because it was common among soldiers in the trenches).

All of these miseries <u>can</u> be avoided (including just plain old tooth decay) by proper brushing of the teeth and gums and even the tongue, plus a good diet (including plenty of Vitamin C). All tooth and gum diseases are caused by an accumulation of bacterial colonies. You might call it a compost pit in your mouth, which soon begins to compost your teeth, too. This can be avoided if you break up those bacterial colonies just once every 24 hours. Many dentists are now becoming more conscious of dental care as preventative medicine. There is a new technique for brushing the teeth once a day which emphasizes a thorough massage of the gums. Using dental floss is also important because the brush can't reach <u>between</u> the teeth. Combined with a good diet, this method is very effective in preventing gum diseases and tooth decay. (See Centerfold for dietary guidelines.) If your gums are red and swollen, or if they bleed when you brush your teeth, see a good dentist and don't be ashamed to learn a new way to brush your teeth -- and keep them!

If you do have gum problems, here are some home remedies you might try:

1. HYDROGEN PEROXIDE RINSE: Combine ¼ cup hydrogen peroxide and ¼ cup water -- rinse mouth and swish through teeth 3 times, 3 times a day, for 5 days. Excellent for bleeding gums, sores in the mouth, trenchmouth.

2. GOLDEN SEAL AND MYRRH: Combine equal parts golden seal powder and myrrh powder and use this to brush the teeth and gums, 3 or 4 times a day. It tastes bitter, but it will do wonders to strengthen the gums.

Please See Also Page 17, Babies and Small Children: Problems & Diet.

asthma

Many things can be done to provide relief for the person who is suffering from asthma; many people have found that they can prevent attacks from occuring entirely. Fresh air is necessary for the lungs to function properly, but warmth is also essential. In Winter, keep the window open a crack, but keep the termperature at about 68 degrees. Walking outdoors in the fresh air is advisable at least once a day; on cold days, dress warm. A vaporizer is very helpful to asthmatics, especially when 1 teaspoon of eucalyptus oil (available at most drugstores) is added per gallon of water. The best kind of vaporizer, to avoid over-heating (also recommended by the Consumer's Guide) is a Cold Vaporizer, or Humidifier. The eucalyptus oil can be added directly to the water, but the filter should be cleaned after each use. This provides wonderful relief, especially when used at night, at the first sign of congestion.

The following is a beneficial tea to use as PREVENTATIVE MEDICINE. Many people who tend to get asthma have strengthened their resistance by drinking 2-3 cups daily. (It's a good idea to make a large pot, and refrigerate it for use as needed.)

Comfrey and Lobelia Tea:
Boil 3 cups of water -- add 2 tsp. comfrey root -- simmer 20 minutes -- remove from heat and add 1½ tsp. lobelia (naturopaths use lobelia for asthma because it relaxes the alveoli -- the tiny air sacs within in lungs) and 2 tsp. peppermint. Cover pot and let sit for 5 minutes.

An effective syrup to use AT THE BEGINNING OF OR DURING AN ATTACK, which alleviates discomfort by dilating the bronchicles (the same thing more powerful medications do, but with less of the uncomfortable side effects) is made with **Ephedra Tea** (also known as Desert Tea, Mormon Tea, and Ma Huang. Chinese Ephedra (Ma Huang) is said to be stronger than American Ephedra, so substitute 3/4 tsp. Ma Huang for 1 tsp. regular Ephedra.)

Ephedra is a natural stimulant, and can increase the heart-beat considerably. Children can be given ephedra, but someone should monitor their heart-beat about a half hour after taking the syrup. (This can be done by holding the child calmly in your lap, with your hand over her/his heart, and counting the heart-beats for 30 seconds, then multiplying it by two. Average pulsations in children over seven are 80-90, one to seven years 80-120, infants 110-130, at birth 130-160.) Catnip is combined with the ephedra to provide a calming counter-effect. If the child's pulse exceeds the average by more than 10 beats, then further sedation is needed. See page 34 on Nervous Tension.

Ephedra Syrup:
Boil 2 cups of water -- add 4 heaping tablespoons ephedra twigs or 3 heaping tablespoons granulated ephedra -- simmer 20 minutes -- remove from heat -- add 2 tablespoons catnip. Brew in covered pot for 5 more minutes. Dose: babies take 3 or 4 eyedroppers; small children take 1-2 teaspoons, adults take 3-4 teaspoons. Wait at least 1/2 hour before considering taking more. This is a very potent syrup, and should be used with care.

continued on next page

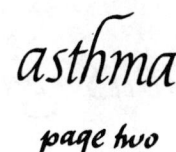

asthma
page two

A standard medication, which has a similar effect, is MARAX SYRUP -- available by prescription. It contains hydroxyzine hydrochloride, ephedrine sulphate, and theophylline. Some people have found that it has less unpleasant side effects than other common medications for asthma. It works best when taken at the first sign of a wheeze.

Another simple method which has helped many people is to carry around a cube of sugar and some EUCALYPTUS OIL. When you have difficulty breathing, put a drop of the oil on the cube of sugar and swallow it.

One of the dangers of wheezing is that you may become DEHYDRATED. To prevent this, try to get at least 4 or 5 cups of fluid every day. An excellent tea for asthmatics, which can help you to regain your strength and your breath is the following Lung Tea. It is difficult to make, so it's worthwhile to make it in large quantities and then refrigerate for use as needed. Try to drink around 4 or 5 cups a day. (if any of these herbs cannot be obtained, they can be omitted.)

LUNG TEA:
a) Boil 12 cups of water. Add
   2 Tbsp. comfrey root
b) simmer 10 minutes, then add
   2 tsp. mullein
   2 tsp. coltsfoot
c) simmer 10 minutes, then remove from heat and add
   2 tsp. corn silk
   4 tsp. lobelia
   3 tsp. red clover
   3 tsp. peppermint

Brew for 5 minutes. Strain. Add as much honey as you want. If this tea is prepared frequently, it is much easier to combine the herbs of parts b and c separately, in large quantities, and then use 2 Tbsp. of the b mix and 5 Tbsp. of the c mix.

LUNG MASSAGE:
if you feel an attack coming on -- or just to strengthen the lungs generally -- it is very useful to firmly scratch or massage the skin along the acupuncture meridian of the lung, starting from the shoulder joint and going down to the outside of the thumb. This is an excellent method to use on children.

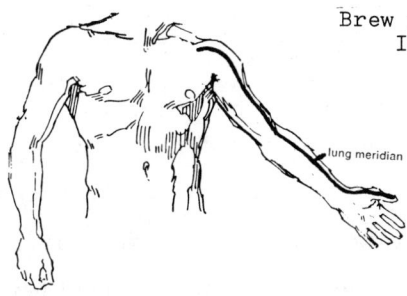

LUNG MERIDIAN

babies & small children: problems & diet

colic

Colic is an attack of abdominal pain caused by spasmodic contractions of the intestine, most common in the first 3 months of life. Many people believe that it is caused by gas. This may come about if the baby swallows too much air, drinks too fast or too much, gets overexcited, or if the mother is very anxious or easily disturbed. It is often helpful to provide a quiet, secure environment for both mother and child, before and at feeding time.

To relieve a colicky baby, the old bounce-n-pat technique is usually the most reliable. Bounce 'em on your knee or pat 'em on your shoulder or do whatever you can to hypnotize them and make them forget all about it. Try giving them a little warm water, too.

Here's an excellent recipe for gas, which works wonders for colic, too:

SLIPPERY ELM TEA: boil 2 cups of water -- sprinkle in 1 tsp. slippery elm powder (granulated is fine, too) -- simmer 20 minutes -- strain -- add honey as desired. Drink as needed.
Note: slippery elm also has a mild laxative effect.

cradle cap

This is an oily yellowish crust that sometimes appears on the scalp of nursing babies, and is caused by excessive secretion of the sebaceous glands in the scalp. All you have to do is put wheat germ oil or vegetable oil on the baby's scalp, leave it on overnight, and the next morning scratch off the softened crust. Then wash the baby's head with shampoo. If you shampoo the hair weekly, it probably won't return, but if it does, just repeat the same treatment.

diaper rash

There are two factors to consider here --

1) The Diapers: many babies are easily irritated by paper diapers and/or rubber pants. If baby has a diaper rash, try cloth diapers without rubber pants at least until it clears up. Better yet, let em run naked if you can. If you're already using cloth diapers, make sure you're using a gentle, non-burning detergent like Ivory. Also be sure to avoid ammonia or bleach. If you want nice, white diapers, hang them in the sun to dry (if there is any). If necessary, use two rinses for the diapers, and/or add a Tablespoon of vinegar to the rinse water.

2) The Baby: it's a good idea to run his or her bottom under some clean water after every change of diapers.

<u>for raw & tender skin</u> -- just dust on plain corn starch. It's cheaper than the commercial stuff, and works just fine.

<u>for dry, chapped skin</u> -- rub in some A&D ointment, or wheat germ oil, or vaseline.

If the rash is <u>really persistent</u>, one of the best methods of treatment is exposure to the sun. Families with babies who have very sensitive skin might even want to invest in a sunlamp (also an excellent way to get your daily vitamin D in sunless places like Seattle). Put the baby's bottom about three feet under the lamp, and keep it there for three minutes, two or three times a day. You should see immediate improvement. Be sure to shade the baby's eyes.

If none of these things work, see your pediatrician; your baby may have a yeast infection or some other special problem.

babies & small children

foreskin ~ infection or irritation of

In England, parents are taught not to pull the foreskin back, as this is believed to be a primary source of infection. They explain that there is a membrane that adheres to the head of the penis. This is a protection against bacteria and should be left intact. At the penis grows, the membrane thins out and gradually tears away from the head. By the time the child is 18 months to 2 years, this membrane should be completely dissolved away, and the foreskin will move easily back and forth. Very rarely this doesn't happen, and then medical assistance may be required to remove the membrane. Many Canadian doctors also agree that it does more harm than good to pull back the foreskin.

In any case, it sometimes happens that at around 2 years old, a child's urine will become very acidic and therefore irritating. It helps to get him to drink water, which dilutes the acid. However, if the foreskin becomes swollen, painful, or even oozy, it will usually respond to this simple treatment:

CORNSTARCH SOAK: dilute 1 Tbsp. cornstarch in $\frac{1}{4}$ cup warm water. Soak a cloth in this solution, then hold it up to the foreskin for about 3 minutes. Repeat 3 times a day. The swelling usually goes down the first day, and goes away in a day or two. (You can buy cornstarch in any supermarket.)

teething

The following methods can be used to relieve the pain of teething:

1. VITAMIN C: Cutting teeth puts so much strain on the body that huge amounts of Vitamin C are used up very quickly, leaving the gums in a weakened condition, which adds considerably to the pain. One of the prime symptoms of Vitamin C dificiency is inflammed gums. Children who are teething can take as much as 500-1000 mg. of Vitamin C, 1-3 times a day. If they're feverish, they can take 250 mg. or more every 2 hours. Powdered ascorbic acid is easy to dissolve in liquid and can then be given by dropper or by bottle.

2. HYLAND'S TEETHING TABLETS: This is a favorite among naturopathic and homeopathic physicians. Each tablet contains Lime Phosphate, Chamomilla, Coffea, and Belladonna (0.000003% alkaloids). Instructions are given on the bottle. Teething Tablets are available at some health food stores, or may be ordered from Standard Homeopathic Company, P.O. Box 61067, Los Angeles, California 90061.

3. SALT: Rub a little salt on their gums.

4. LOCAL COMMERCIAL ANAESTHETICS: Anbesol or Chloraseptic (available in most drugstores) usually work nicely.

5. ALCOHOL: if all else fails, take a shot of wine or brandy or whisky. It's traditional. Rub it on the kid's gums, even. But don't give too much to the baby, because not all infants can tolerate alcohol. And it is habit-forming. It may be better for both of you to just take some catnip tea, or Calms Forte (see page 34 on Nervous Tension).

food for infants

A good time to offer food to your baby is when he/she begins to show an interest in it. But be careful to introduce foods one by one, waiting a few days after each new food to see if there's any possible allergic reaction to it. Beware of the common misconception that tooth decay can be avoided by substituting honey and dried fruit for white sugar. These foods are sticky, and if you're not brushing your baby's teeth, they're as good a medium as sugar for decay. Also, if you start your baby on vegetables, plain yogurt, and unsweetened teas -- then as they grow older they often retain a taste for such foods. Little ones often like milk or yogurt with brewer's yeast and a little molasses; start them on it while they're very young. On the other hand, if you start them out with fruits and sweetened foods, they're likely to get a sweet tooth and often will not be inclined to eat vegetables when they get older. Surveys have borne out these theories.

strong teeth & bones

If you child seems particularly susceptible to tooth decay, even though her/his diet seems adequate, there may be a genetic tendency toward soft teeth and/or bones. To counteract this, you may want to supplement their diet with:

1. CALCIUM: Most health food stores carry a liquid form of calcium. See page 58.
2. VITAMINS A & D: These can also be given in drops.
3. VITAMIN C: Children love acerola pills and will gladly take 100 mg.s per day.

constipation

This is usually due to a dietary deficiency, or eating too fast, not chewing your food thoroughly (chewing produces saliva, which aids digestion), or from tension, etc.

dietary suggestions:

1. GREENS: eat plenty of greens, especially raw ones -- they put roughage in your diet.
2. OIL: substitute vegetable oils for animal fats. Try soy, safflower, or peanut oil. (All-Blend Oil, at health food stores, is excellent.)
3. YOGURT: eat plenty of yogurt or acidophilus, preferably a brand like Continental. Yogurt restores beneficial intestinal bacteria.
4. BREWER'S YEAST: take 1-3 Tbsp.s of brewer's yeast or torula yeast a day. See recipes pg. 43.
5. FRUIT: try an all-fruit diet at least one day a week. Raw fruits are especially helpful.
6. WATER: drink plenty of water. Constipation is often caused by dehydration. Try 1 cup of hot water before bed.

BULK & ROUGHAGE: Eat whole, unprocessed grains, whole fruits (with skins), leafy vegetables, raw carrots, whole cereals and grains.

PAY ATTENTION TO YOUR BODY: When you have the urge to go to the bathroom, take advantage of it.

ways to deal with the symptoms:

Try ONE of the following.

1. BRAN: Bran has the capacity to absorb moisture, so when it's taken with plenty of liquid, it swells up and forms a soft mass that passes easily through the intestines. Take 2 Tbsp. or up to 1 cup of crude bran per day. Mix with juice or cereal or with yogurt and molasses. Always drink 1-2 cups of liquid at the same time. (Packaged and processed bran cereals contain less fibre content and none of the moisture-absorbing properties of crude bran.)

2. HERB-LAX: These are pills which contain strong laxative and anti-gas herbs. The effective is powerful, without griping or painful gas. Try one tablet before bed. If this is not adequate, try 2 tablets the following night. Increase as needed, but discontinue when the desired effect is achieved. Contains senna, buckthorn bark, licorice root, alfalfa, fennel seed, anise seed, blue melva flower, culver root, rhubarb root, and jalap root. Herb-Lax is available from Shaklee distributors. Look in the yellow pages of your phone book, under Health Food Products or Cleaning Products (they sell both).

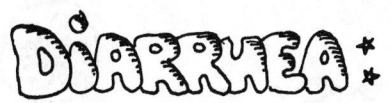

DIARRHEA *

If you have the runs, it's a good idea to consider the following: Maybe your diet is not right; you may be getting too little protein, or eating too many soybeans. If you're vegetarian, and your protein intake might be deficient, get a copy of DIET FOR A SMALL PLANET (see last page for list of Books). Or maybe you're eating too much too fast.

If the following remedies don't work, see a doctor and have a stool test taken. You may have some form of dysentery that should be dealt with right away.

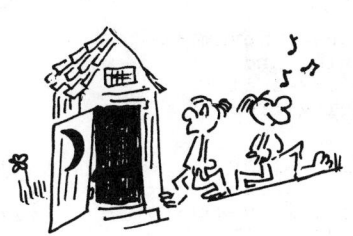

1. Try fasting for 36 hours (a night, a day, and a night. Drink only liquids and avoid milk or milk products, sweetened fruit juices, and honey. Drink spring water if you can. Get plenty of fluids. Nourishing teas (separately or together) for diarrhea include:
   comfrey
   blackberry root
   ginger root (fresh grated is best)
(simmer the above for 20 minutes -- one tsp. per cup of water)
   mullein
   nettle
(simmer the above for 10 minutes -- one tsp. per cup of water)
   peppermint
   elder flowers
(brew these for 5 minutes -- cover one tsp. herbs with one cup boiling water)

Fasting is recommended because it allows your system to cleanse itself. An infection often breaks off the brush border on the villae of the small intestines -- which means your body can't absorb carbohydrates. If you fast for 36 hours, you allow the brush border to grow back. Babies and small children often fast spontaneously; they should be allowed to do this. It's a safe method for babies, but if vomiting also occurs -- especially in babies under 3 months -- be sure to consult a doctor, because dehydration could occur and could even be fatal.

2. Cinnamon and cayenne tea: bring 2 cups of water to a boil; add $\frac{1}{4}$ tsp. cinnamon (1/8 tsp. for babies) and a dash of cayenne pepper and simmer for 20 minutes. Cool, strain, and take a few sips, as needed. Usually tightens the bowels immediately.

3. Apple cider vinegar and honey: take 1 tablespoon of apple cider vinegar and 1 tablespoon of honey in a glass of hot water, 3 times a day.

See also page 8 on Belly-Aches.

Note: The enzyme lactase enables one to digest milk. But many people lack this enzyme, including the majority of American blacks, many third-world people, and some Caucasians. A lack of this enzyme can cause severe diarrhea after drinking milk.

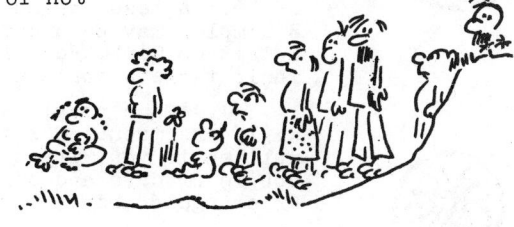

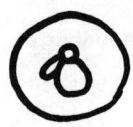

HEMORRHOIDS

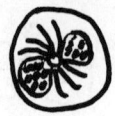
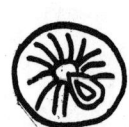

Hemorrhoids are usually connected with constipation, so if you have this trouble, you may also want to see page 18 on Constipation.

The following remedies have been very helpful:

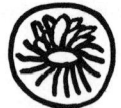

   1. CLEANLINESS: After each bowel movement and after wiping, dip a Q-Tip in water and insert into the anus (bearing down makes it easier to insert). Repeat this, using fresh Q-Tips, until it comes out clean.

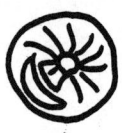

   2. LEMON JUICE OR WITCH HAZEL: After cleaning as described above, dip a fresh Q-Tip into lemon juice (bottled lemon juice is available in grocery stores) or witch hazel (bottled witch hazel is available in drugstores), and again insert into the anus. This may cause a burning sensation, but it goes away quickly and then the itching is relieved. If the burning is uncomfortable, then plain water may again be applied.

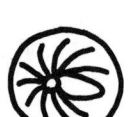
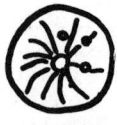

   3. VITAMIN B6: A deficiency of this vitamin can cause hemorrhoids. B6 is part of the B Complex, which should always be taken as a complete complex (see page 54), so I suggest taking a form of B Complex which contains 10 mg. of B6, 3 times a day after each meal, or take a B Complex tablet that contains 25-50 mg. of B6 once a day. Usually 3-14 days is enough to get rid of hemorrhoids, depending on how serious they are. I suggest stopping the vitamin when the hemorrhoids are gone, but beginning it again whenever you're under a lot of stress (which uses up B vitamins), or whenever you begin to feel the first signs of a new hemorrhoid. (Plus Formula 71 B Complex with C is good. It contains 10 mg. of B6. A less expensive and more potent Balanced B Complex may be ordered from the Wholesale Nutrition Club, Box 1113, Sunnyvale, Ca. 94088. Their tablets contain 50 mg. of B6.)

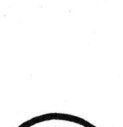
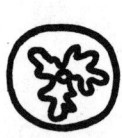

   4. Some people who take brewer's yeast daily are troubled with an itchy anus. If this applies to you, try stopping the yeast for a couple of days and see if the itching goes away. Or change brands.

NOTE: an itchy anus may also be caused by pinworms. See page 21.

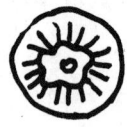

PINWORMS:

Many people have pinworms and don't realize it. An itchy anus is the most common symptom, particularly if the itchiness becomes most intense at night and around the full moon, because during these times the worms become move active and come out to lay their eggs (this may sound bizarre, but recent studies of eels show that they have a similar response to the moon). Pinworms will not necessarily show up in the feces. The test for pinworms is taken just by wrapping a piece of scotch tape around your finger, sticky side out, and touching it to the opening of your anus. If there are any eggs there, they will adhere to the tape. Then the tape is put onto a slide, sticky side down, and examined under a microscope. One doctor we know has her patients do this 3 mornings in a row, at 5 a.m. each morning, because she says the worms are most active at this time. One random test, taken any time of the day or the month may be enough to give you a positive result, but a negative from one test may not necessarily be reliable.

Pinworms become most numerous when there is also constipation, in which case they are like earthworms in a compost heap. If you are constipated, be sure to treat that, too. (See page 18 on Constipation.)

Some nutritionists think that people who have a well-balanced diet won't get worms at all. If you have worms, improve your diet to build up resistance. Don't eat sugar while you have worms, because they thrive on it. Also be sure to wash your hands after you use the bathroom, to avoid reinfecting yourself. <u>All members</u> of the household should be tested if one member has them -- pinworms spread very easily.

GARLIC: eat a clove of raw garlic every day for 3 days (see page 3 on garlic). At the end of the third day, take 1 tablet of HERB-LAX (see page 18), or 1 cup of SENNA AND PEPPERMINT TEA: cover ½ tsp. senna leaves and ½ tsp. peppermint leaves (to prevent griping) with 1 cup boiling water. Brew in covered pot for 3-5 minutes. Drink plain or with honey. This should have a laxative effect, to help wash out the worms. But if the bowels do not move very freely, repeat again the following night, and double the dosage. The garlic won't kill the larva, so wait one week until the eggs have hatched, and then repeat the same treatment. Worms can be very stubborn and very difficult to get rid of, so wait one more week and repeat the treatment one more time. The same remedy may be used for children.

When WOMEN have pinworms, they sometimes get into the vagina. These can be drawn out by sitting in a pot of hot water (a sitz bath) with 1½ cups of EPSOM SALT per gallon of water used. Do this twice a day for 3 days. Also apply ZINC OXIDE (available by prescription) to the vaginal opening, the opening of the anus, and the area in between.

PINWORMS (also called THREADWORMS) are tiny white worms, a little thicker than thread, and around ½ inch long.

hepatitis

prevention

If exposed to hepatitis -- that is, if you've had close contact with someone who has infectious hepatitis -- during the 2 weeks before or a few days after the jaundice (yellow discoloration of the skin due to liver dysfunction) begins -- then you should:

1. Get a gamma globulin shot. This may not definitely prevent the disease, but it will make it milder if you do get it. Gamma globulin is produced naturally by the body when it gets attacked by any foreign substance and, according to Adelle Davis, the body produces an excess of its own gamma globulin if you eat an excessive amount of protein.

2. Isolate infected people while they are jaundiced, and for a week after that. One or two people should get gamma globulin shots and stay with the infected person, or visit them frequently, so that the person with hepatitis will be helped, and the community will not be exposed to this highly contagious disease. Keep plates, cups, silverware etc. in a separate place and wash with a separate cloth or sponge. Sterilize by boiling for 20 minutes. Use separate towels, and soak in a disinfectant (lysol, bleach) before washing the towel. Watch out for things like everybody's toothbrush in the same glass. EACH PERSON SHOULD WASH THE TOILET SEAT WITH LYSOL AFTER USING IT, AND WASH THEIR HANDS VERY CAREFULLY WITH BETADINE OR SOME OTHER DISINFECTANT AFTER USING THE TOILET (hepatitis is spread through the feces, so this is particularly important).

3. As always: good nutrition (especially lots of protein) is the best prevention.

cause

There are technically two kinds of hepatitis:

INFECTIOUS HEPATITIS -- believed to be passed through the feces, the blood (so be sure to bandage all wounds), or the water.

SERUM HEPATITIS -- less common, it is usually associated with dirty needles; it's somewhat more serious and can last much longer.

Recovery from hepatitis is slow; from 1 to 4 months to return to normal, with infectious hep, though small children can have it for as little as 3 days. The more rest you get, and the better your diet, the sooner you'll recover.

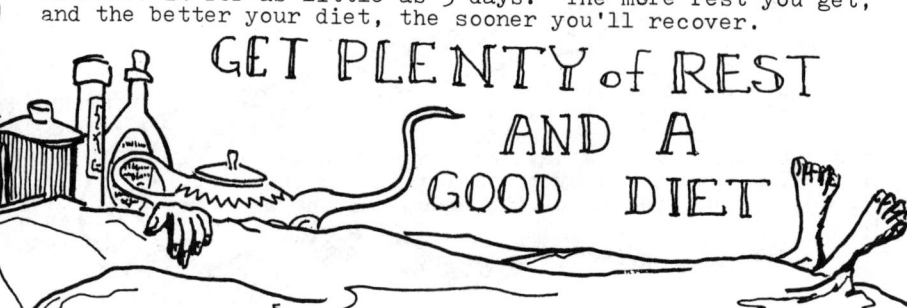

GET PLENTY of REST AND A GOOD DIET

avoid:

The liver will be unable to handle drugs and alcohol for at least 6 months, so be sure to avoid alcohol, barbituates, amphetamines, sulfa drugs, and heroin.

when you need a doctor

hepatitis page two

1. If you've had close contact with someone who has hepatitis, see a doctor to get a gamma globulin shot.
2. If you have some of the signs and symptoms listed below, see a doctor to determine if you definitely do have hepatitis, so that you can isolate yourself and begin following the advice given here. Basically all the doc can do is tell you yep, you got hep, so get lots of rest and eat well.
3. See a doctor again in 6-8 weeks for a follow-up blood test, to tell:
   a. if you are over the disease,
   b. if it has done any permanent damage to your liver, and
   c. if you are a carrier, even though you may feel better yourself.

signs & symptoms

Fever, yellow tint to skin or eyes, fatigue, dark urine, grayish feces, muscle aches, a cold that won't go away, loss of appetite, enlarged tender liver (under rib cage on right side), nausea, loss of taste for cigarettes. A person who is laid up with hepatitis after the jaundice sets in will barely feel strong enough to get up and go to the bathroom.

nutrition

AVOID fried foods and animal fats (the liver is too weak to do its usual job of breaking down fats in the body).

Get plenty of PROTEIN: 100-125 grams a day (see section of Pregnancy, page 44, for foods high in protein).

Get lots of CALORIES: 3000 calories a day. Use honey and molasses freely. But avoid eating food made with a lot of shortening and fats that you can't handle. Vegetable oil is ok. Also good are lots of fruit juices, fruits, malted milk pdr.

LECITHIN should be taken daily. The liver normally produces its own lecithin, which breaks down fats, but during hepatitis many liver cells are destroyed and the body loses its ability to process fats.

To help rebuild your body, the following vitamins may be used:

VITAMIN C: 250-500 mgs., 4 times a day (Such large quantities of Vitamin C may produce a calcium deficiency, so be sure to also take the Sorcerer's Potion described on the next page, or see page 58 on sources of Calcium.

VITAMIN B COMPLEX: Plus Products Formula 71 is excellent -- use as directed on the bottle.

VITAMIN A: 5000 - 10,000 Units daily

VITAMIN E: 100 Units daily

herbs

GOLDEN SEAL ROOT POWDER: helps detoxify the liver. Take one 00 cap (1/4 tsp.) followed by warm water, 1-3 times a day.

HEPATITIS TEA: This tea is especially important for vegetarians who don't want to use the Sorcerer's Potion described on the next page.

Boil 10 cups of water. Add:
    2 Tbsp. dandelion root
    2 Tbsp. burdock root
    2 Tbsp. yellow dock root
Simmer 10 minutes. Then add:
    2 Tbsp. stinging nettle
Simmer 10 minutes. Remove from heat. Then add:
    2 Tbsp. red clover
    2 Tbsp. alfalfa
    2 Tbsp. peppermint

Try to drink 5-6 cups per day. If there is nausea and vomiting, add 2 Tbsp. slippery elm at the same time you add the dandelion. Also eat plenty of dark green leafy vegetables. Steamed greens are easiest to digest, and steamed comfrey leaves are excellent.

hepatitis

When you're very sick, during the first few days, you should stay in bed and have someone take care of you. At first, you'll probably feel nauseous and unable to eat. Try to at least drink the Sorcerer's Potion, as described below. It will supply your total nutritional needs. It will provide <u>all</u> the elements necessary for optimal cell regeneration, in the right form, at the right site, and at the same time. This is vital in regenerating cells to rebuild the damaged liver. <u>All</u> factors must be present in order for cell-building to take place. The Milk/Grain Mix "predigests" protein, which the liver would do if it was healthy; also lecithin does the bile's job of breaking down big fat globules. In hepatitis the usual bile flow is disrupted due to damage to the liver.

If you've been exposed to hep, drink two cups of Sorcerer's Potion a day as good preventative medicine -- especially if you can't get a gamma globulin shot. If you have hep and can't eat anything else, one quart of this a day supplies all your needed nutrients. Even when you do begin to eat solid food, continue to drink one to two cups a day for 60 days after symptoms disappear, in order to insure complete recovery.

SORCERERS POTION

(thank you, Adelle Davis)

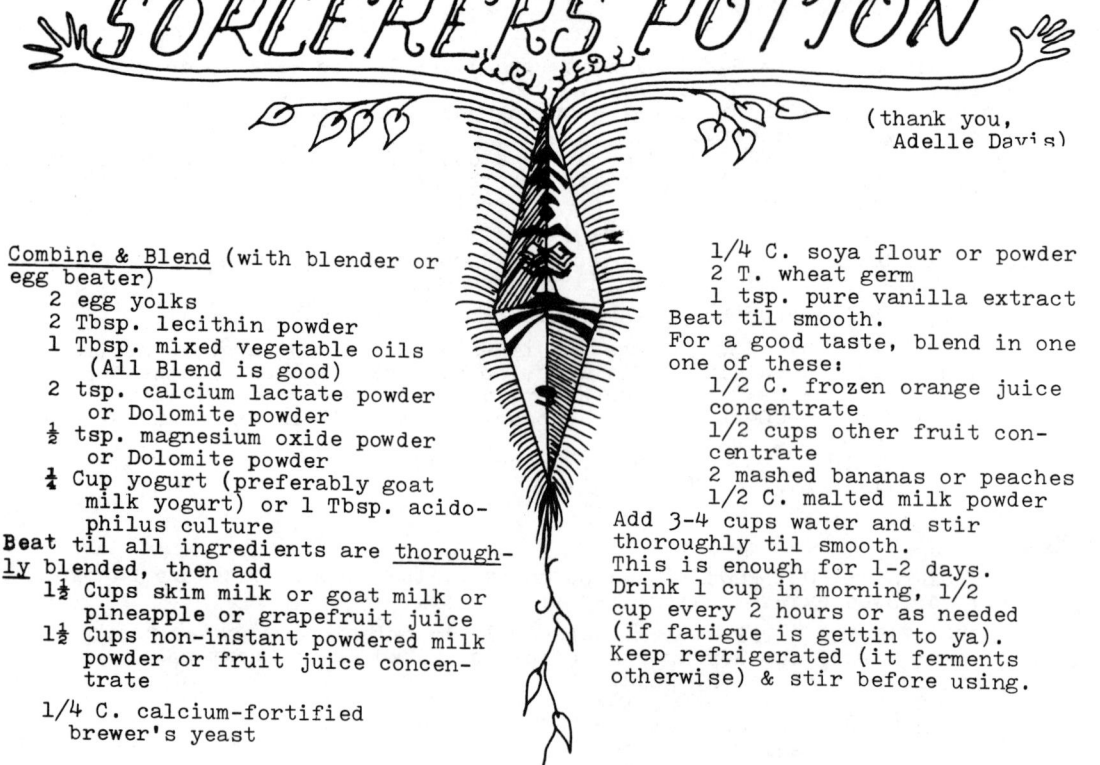

<u>Combine & Blend</u> (with blender or egg beater)
- 2 egg yolks
- 2 Tbsp. lecithin powder
- 1 Tbsp. mixed vegetable oils (All Blend is good)
- 2 tsp. calcium lactate powder or Dolomite powder
- ½ tsp. magnesium oxide powder or Dolomite powder
- ¼ Cup yogurt (preferably goat milk yogurt) or 1 Tbsp. acidophilus culture

<u>Beat</u> til all ingredients are <u>thoroughly</u> blended, then add
- 1½ Cups skim milk or goat milk or pineapple or grapefruit juice
- 1½ Cups non-instant powdered milk powder or fruit juice concentrate
- 1/4 C. calcium-fortified brewer's yeast
- 1/4 C. soya flour or powder
- 2 T. wheat germ
- 1 tsp. pure vanilla extract

Beat til smooth.

For a good taste, blend in one one of these:
- 1/2 C. frozen orange juice concentrate
- 1/2 cups other fruit concentrate
- 2 mashed bananas or peaches
- 1/2 C. malted milk powder

Add 3-4 cups water and stir thoroughly til smooth. This is enough for 1-2 days. Drink 1 cup in morning, 1/2 cup every 2 hours or as needed (if fatigue is gettin to ya). Keep refrigerated (it ferments otherwise) & stir before using.

hair

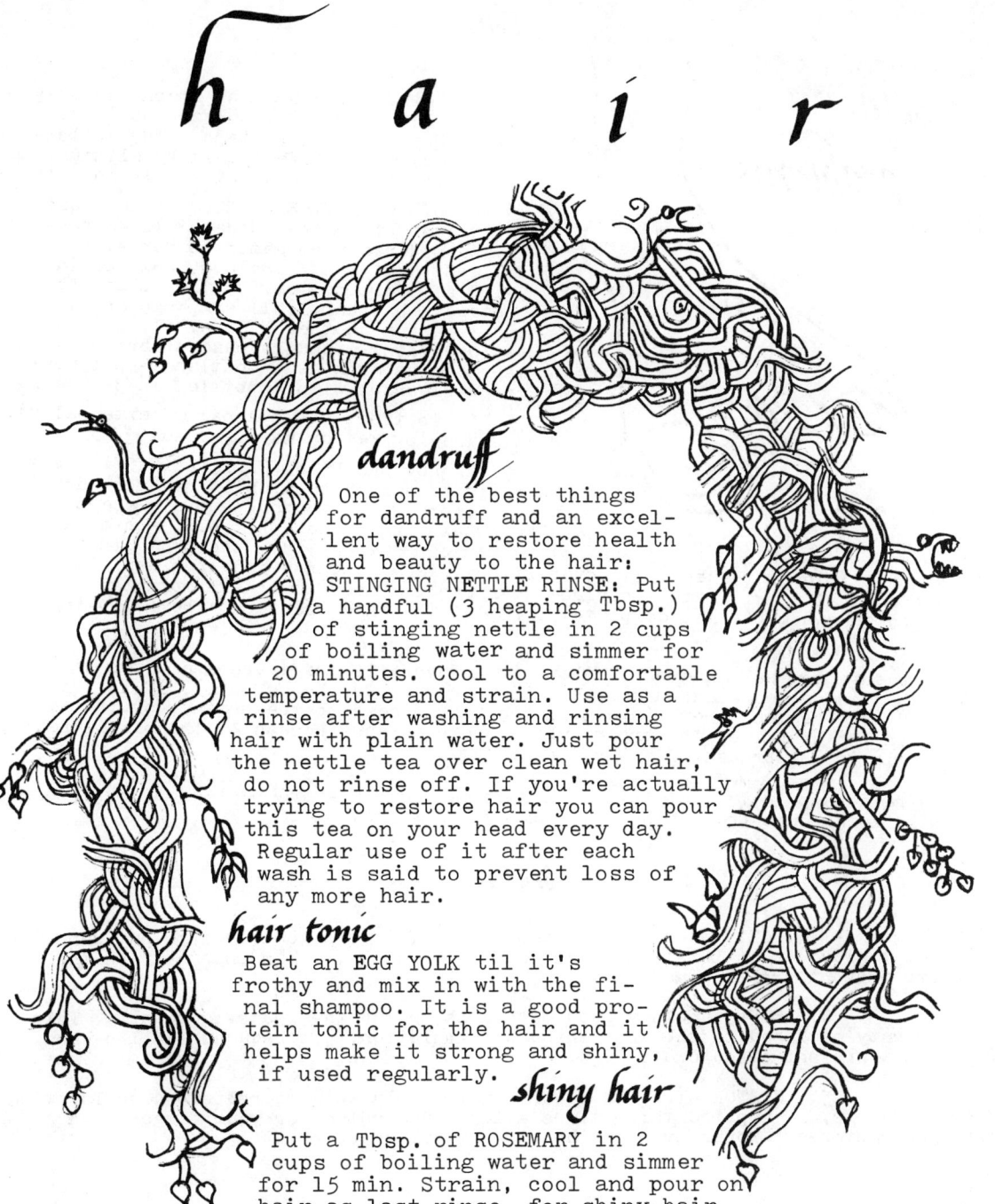

dandruff

One of the best things for dandruff and an excellent way to restore health and beauty to the hair: STINGING NETTLE RINSE: Put a handful (3 heaping Tbsp.) of stinging nettle in 2 cups of boiling water and simmer for 20 minutes. Cool to a comfortable temperature and strain. Use as a rinse after washing and rinsing hair with plain water. Just pour the nettle tea over clean wet hair, do not rinse off. If you're actually trying to restore hair you can pour this tea on your head every day. Regular use of it after each wash is said to prevent loss of any more hair.

hair tonic

Beat an EGG YOLK til it's frothy and mix in with the final shampoo. It is a good protein tonic for the hair and it helps make it strong and shiny, if used regularly.

shiny hair

Put a Tbsp. of ROSEMARY in 2 cups of boiling water and simmer for 15 min. Strain, cool and pour on hair as last rinse, for shiny hair.

skin problems

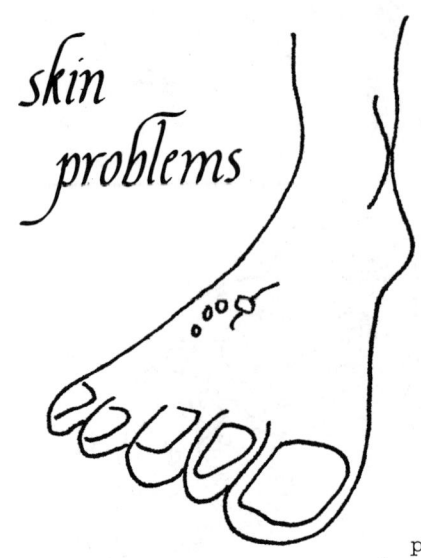

boils

Boils are caused by staph, so they tend to keep recurring unless you do something to clear up the staph. The following remedy works effectively by eliminating the staph, so that new boils will not form.

OIL OF BITTER ORANGE: take 4 drops in a glass of orange juice, 3 times a day. May be ordered from Nature's Herbs, 281 Ellis Street, San Francisco, California 94102 at 50¢ per $\frac{1}{4}$ oz. bottle, plus 25¢ postage. Use until all symptoms are gone, and then for another 3 days. If it's a serious, long-standing case of boils, you may need as much as 3 bottles -- but most cases clear up with 1 bottle, in 3-7 days.

To treat boils locally (externally), this drawing remedy may be used:

HOT BREAD AND MILK POULTICE: white bread is preferred because it has more drawing power. Before going to bed, cut a piece of bread somewhat larger than the boil -- heat a small amount of milk until it's as hot as you can stand -- dip the bread in the milk and put it over the boil -- cover with a piece of gauze and then wrap it with adhesive so that it will stay in place overnight. Remove the next morning. If it has helped somewhat but not completely, repeat the same treatment the following night.

NOTE: Be sure to see a doctor if there is a fever, if there are a cluster of boils (this is called a carbuncle, and is more serious than a boil), if the boil is in the head region (where infection has easy access to the brain), or if the boil is in the armpit or the groin (where there is easy access to the bloodstream), or if it is in the breast of a nursing mother.

Previous printings of this book recommended a mustard paste for boils, but one child got a burn from using this remedy, so we now omit it.

bruises

1. ICE: whenever you bop yourself it's a good idea to put some ice on it right away, or at least run real cold water on it. This anesthetizes the area and helps prevent swelling and bruising.

2. RUB: another good method is to rub the spot vigorously. This brings plenty of blood to the area through stimulation. It reduces swelling and often helps prevent discoloration.

3. CASTOR OIL: this works remarkably well to relieve discoloration after it occurs, if applied three times a day. Use cotton or your fingers. Available in drugstores. Works even in the case of "black eyes".

eczema & psoriasis

skin problems
page two

Use all of the following, for 2 weeks:
   COD LIVER OIL: 2 Tbsp. per day
   SESAME OIL: 1 tsp., uncooked, per day. May be used on salads.
   CRANBERRY JUICE: 3 cups per day, any form (Ocean Spray is okay).
   Externally, use one of the following:
      ALOE VERA: (see below)
      COMFREY OINTMENT: Available in health food stores and co-ops.
After 2 weeks, the condition should be significantly improved. Continue to drink 1 cup of cranberry juice per day, preventatively. Repeat the whole regime if a new outbreak occurs. Don't use cod liver oil for more than 2 weeks at a time.

burns

   ICE: Cold water or ice should be applied to burns immediately until the burning sensation stops.
   NOTE: <u>If the burn is serious</u>, consult a First Aid Manual and/or a doctor. Consider treating for shock (elevate legs, maintain body temperature with blankets). Give fluids if the patient is conscious.

HOME REMEDIES FOR BURNS

1) ALOE VERA: This succulent plant yields an excellent ointment for all kinds of burns. Cut off a piece of the lower leaf of the plant (so that it will continue to put out new upper leaves), peel back the outer skin, and apply the thick jelly directly to the burn. In most cases, the effect is immediate: the redness can literally be seen going away and the pain eases at once. It can be used effectively for chemical burns as well as ordinary burns, and I've also heard that it's effective for radiation burns. The gel is bottled and sold, but it's less effective than when taken directly from the plant. Consult your local nursery for where to obtain an aloe vera plant. Aloe is a succulent, grows in direct sunlight, and needs watering only once every 7-10 days.
   2) HONEY may be applied to burns. It soothes and is soon absorbed by the skin. Cover with gauze if you want a cover on it.
   3) WHEAT GERM OIL or VITAMIN E: open Vitamin E capsule by putting a pin through both ends -- either one may be applied directly.
   4) CALENDULA CERATE: a homeopathic salve made of pot marigold flowers in a bland base -- works just beautifully on burns. Also good for chapping, dryness, diaper rash. A one-ounce tube may be ordered from Standard Homeopathic Company, P.O. Box 61067, Los Angeles, California. A tube lasts a long time. This is my favorite remedy for burns.

skin problems

page three

staph infections

Staphylococcus is a spherical-shaped bacteria which causes pus-filled infections in wounds. It's very common in country communes, particularly those that have no refrigeration. This may be due to the fact that when meat and dairy products are stored without refrigeration or left out overnight, germs get into the food, multiply rapidly, and secrete a poisonous toxin which is not destroyed by heating or cooking. This is especially true if the food is not well covered. A protein deficiency increases susceptibility to this bacteria -- which makes it all the more common in vegetarian groups and communes that are trying to live at a subsistence level. Another factor is cleanliness. Keeping clean can help prevent staph in the first place. Staph is common in people who are deficient in Vitamin B complex (a lot of vegetarians have this deficiency). See page on vitamins. Once again, in order to cure staph it is necessary to treat both internally and externally. If it doesn't work, be sure to see a doctor.

external treatment

Prepare a mixture of 1 tsp. powdered myrrh, 1 tsp. powdered golden seal, ½ tsp. cayenne -- boil gently in two cups of water for 20 minutes. Soak the infected area for at least 10 minutes, keeping the water as hot as possible to draw out the infection. Then dry well and apply a paste of golden seal and water to the area; then bandage.

internal treatment

Take 250-1000 mgs. of Vitamin C, 3 times a day, to detoxify the body. Drink juices and teas freely. In addition, use one or both of these remedies:

1. OIL OF BITTER ORANGE: take 4 drops in a glass of orange juice, 3 times a day. May be ordered from Nature's Herbs, 281 Ellis Street, San Francisco, California 94102. Use until all symptoms are gone, and then for another 3 days. This is extremely effective for staph.

2. ECHINACEA & BURDOCK TEA: Boil 4 cups of water, add 2 tsps. echinacea root and 2 tsps. burdock root -- simmer 20 minutes -- drink 3 cups a day until all symptoms are gone, and then for another 3 days.

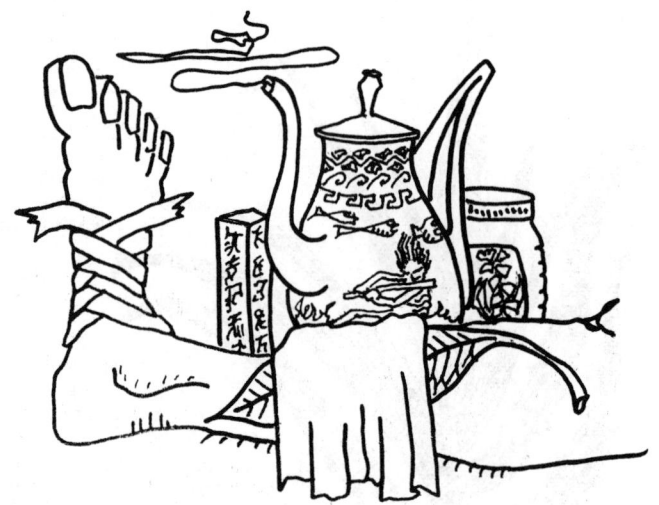

pubic area ~ itching

genital itching

First, make sure you're not wearing any kind of clothing which would irritate this area, such as nylon underpants, which keep the moisture in and the air out. Cotton is fine. Simple remedies for itching of the vulva, the genitals, the area between the legs, heat rash -- for both men and women:

1. SLIPPERY ELM INFUSION - Bring 1 cup of water to a boil, add 2 tsps. slippery elm powder and simmer gently for 20 minutes. Let cool and apply to area with fingers or with cotton.
2. CORN STARCH - Sprinkle liberally over itching area.
3. BUTTERMILK - Apply to itching area with fingers or with cotton.

pubic hair itching

Sometimes the pubic hair, like the hair on our heads, itches -- not from lice, but from dryness or whatever. Make sure you don't have crabs by looking very closely at the roots of the hair follicles for tiny white or transparent creatures which, when pulled away, look like microscopic crabs. Look also for eggs, which are mere specks the size of a pin-point and cling tenaciously to the hairs. If you have crabs, use Pyrinate A 200, which is available in drugstores.

If you haven't got crabs, but you do have an itch, here are some things you can do:

1. STINGING NETTLE
   boil 1 cup of water, add 2 heaping tablespoons of stinging nettle, and simmer for 20 minutes. Let cool and strain. Splash onto area.

2. SLIPPERY ELM INFUSION
   (see above)

3. WHEAT GERM OIL
   apply to area, rubbing it well into hair & skin.

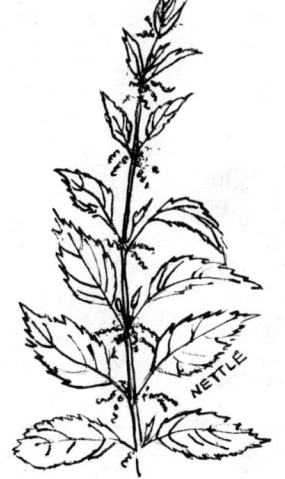
NETTLE

herpes

Herpes are little water-filled vesicles. They're called "cold sores" or canker sores when they occur on the lips; this is now called Herpes Simplex Virus Type 1 and almost always occurs above the waist. The herpes that affects the pubic area is much more severe, and is called Herpes Simplex Virus Type 2. It is a venereal disease, which means simply that it is spread through sexual intercourse -- when the blisters are present. It cannot be urged too strongly that people who have this disease refrain from intercourse while the sores are present. Herpes attacks twice as many people as syphilis, and may soon be as pervasive as gonorrhea.

The herpes virus can live almost indefinitely inside the human body, and so far there is no good way to get rid of it. The blisters appear suddenly -- often in the presence of stress -- and then suddenly go away, within 4 days to a month. But that's not the end of it; a new outbreak may come again, in a few days or a few months. Sometimes it does go away permanently by itself. Since herpes often occurs during times of stress, see also Nervous Tension, page 34.

cancer of the cervix

It has been found that women who have herpes of the cervix are eight times more likely to develop cancer of the cervix than uninfected women. A regular pap smear can determine whether you have herpes of the cervix as well as whether you have cancer of the cervix. Women with herpes should be conscientious about getting a pap test taken every 6 months. Early detection of cancer can make a big difference. Even if you succeed in eliminating the symptoms, there's no guarantee that the inactivated herpes will not continue to cause cancer, so women who have had herpes at any time are urged to get pap tests every 6 months.

internal treatment

VITAMIN C: Massive doses of Vitamin C are the most potent anti-viral treatment. Herpes is a virus. Many people have used the following treatment and have had no recurrences of herpes. Some have had only minor and infrequent occurrences. Take 10 grams (10,000 mgs.) of Vitamin C per day for 10 days. I'd suggest using 2 grams of ascorbic acid powder, 5 times a day. You could take 2 grams of ascorbic acid powder, 5 times per day.

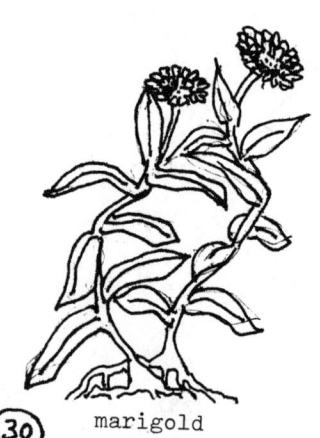

marigold

To increase the effectiveness of this treatment, combine it with a 1-5 day fast. While fasting, drink plenty of fruit juices and the following tea:

BURDOCK ROOT OR SEED TEA: Boil 4 cups of water. Add 1 Tbsp. burdock root or seed. Simmer 20 minutes. After evaporation, this will make 3 cups of tea. Drink 3 cups per day while fasting. Burdock is an excellent blood purifier; it encourages the kidneys and other organs to eliminate toxins from the blood. It's also very good for the skin.

Note: If CONSTIPATION is present, be sure to see and follow the suggestions on page 18. The bowels are one way that the body has to eliminate toxins; if this way is closed, then eruptions will often occur on the skin.

Begin to break your fast slowly, with fruits and vegetables. The next day you can add grain and dairy products, if you like. Wait another day before adding eggs and meat. Go easy on salt, and try to eliminate sugar, white flour, alcohol, caffeine, and tobacco. See pages 32-33 for dietary guidelines.

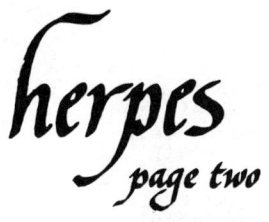

herpes
page two

external treatment

1. CALENDULA TINCTURE: This tincture may be prepared at home, or may be ordered from Standard Homeopathic Company, P.O. Box 61067, Los Angeles, California. Calendula is another name for Pot Marigolds. It contains properties which are extremely beneficial to the skin. For home preparation, pick fresh flowers (heads only) and pack tightly in a glass jar and cover with drinking alcohol. Vodka works well. Shake once a day for 13 days and then strain off the liquid. For best results, most herbalists begin making tinctures at the full moon (which is expansive) and finish just before the new moon. Before using the tincture, dilute with 10 times as much water (the same dilution may be used with the homeopathic tincture). If blisters are active, use as often as desired to relieve itching. You may want to apply it with cotton after each urination (urine does cause itching, if it touches the sores).

2. COTTON UNDERWEAR: Avoid nylon underwear; nylon keeps the air out.

3. SUN LAMP: To build up the flesh and dry out the blisters, place a sun lamp at 18 inches from the area and leave it on for 30 seconds, 4 times a day for 3 days; then for 1 minute 3 times a day for 3 days; and then 2 minutes 3 times a day for 3 days.

4. HOT BATHS: a very hot shallow bath (or a deep one) may be used as often as desired to clean the herpes and help relieve the itching. A hair dryer may be used to dry the sores and give relief.

pregnant women

One of the worst aspects of herpes is that if a pregnant woman has active herpes blisters when she goes into labor, there is one chance in four that her child will die or be seriously damaged. 40-50% are severely brain damaged. Others get hepatitis or jaundice, or herpes skin lesions, or just a fever. The effects are extremely variable.

According to Dr. George Ray at Children's Orthopedic Hospital in Seattle (the only place in Seattle that does herpes cultures), all of the cases he's seen of children whose mothers had herpes were born to women who got their first case of herpes during their last trimester (the last 3 months of pregnancy). For this reason, I strongly suggest having no new sex partner(s) during the last 3 months of pregnancy, and urging your regular partner(s) to do the same. This is <u>especially</u> important for women who've never had herpes, because the first attack of this disease is the most potent.

Herpes is a primary viral infection, often accompanied by a fever, and you can expect to feel extremely weak and sick from it. If you do have these symptoms after a possible exposure to herpes, then see a doctor. The blister may be on the cervix, so it may not be noticeable.

If you already have herpes, and you're pregnant, you should still be careful, especially in you last month. Since herpes are stress-related, do whatever you can to reduce stress and follow these guidelines:

* get plenty of rest
* eat at least 2 Tbsp. yogurt, 3-4 times per day
* have at least 1 tsp. of brewer's yeast per day
* take 1000 mg. or more of Vitamin C (after the first 3 months of pregnancy, it should be safe to use the Vitamin C treatment described above)

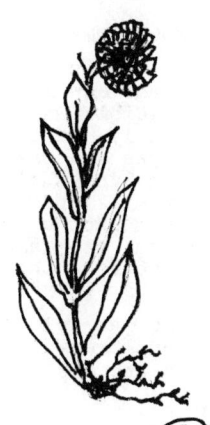

PROVIDING NOURISHMENT

Good guidelines for the provision of nourishment are difficult to find. Need varies with age, sex, lifestyle, work, culture and climate. I believe that each person is a unique chemistry unto themself. So how can I presume to tell you what you should or shouldn't eat? Yet I've found that there are certain guidelines to good health, which seem to apply to almost everyone. In this small space, we can only consider a few issues. I hope to stimulate your interest so you'll look further (if you haven't already). The Book List on page 64 should act as a good jumping-off point.

Good nutrition is central to good health, so we can all benefit from paying full attention to what and how we eat. There's no point in learning how to heal yourself if you haven't paid attention to how to feed yourself. Learning how to prepare foods and how to select foods is vitally important. We cannot be healthy if we eat food that has no vitality. Chemical fertilizers destroy the vitality of the soil. Food grown in such soil lacks some of the vital nutrients for a healthy body. Try to get organic food.

The best way to know what you're eating is to grow it yourself, with compost and manure and mulch. Be sure you're not paying "novelty" prices for basic foods. Find out if there are any co-ops in your area: these stores usually offer high quality food, to members, at reasonable prices. If not, you might want to get together with your neighbors to form a "food conspiracy." This is a tongue-in-cheek expression for a method of distributing food which leaves out the packaging and the middle-man, and results in much cheaper food. It's a neighborhood group which buys food in bulk, and then donates labor to pick up the food and transport it. Members meet at a designated time and place, and pick up and package their own orders. It's a good plan for people who have more time than money, or for people who want to buy in large quantities. For more information, see the Food Conspiracy Cookbook & Members Manual by Lois Wickstrom, available from Spring Books, 1150 St. Paul St., Denver, Colorado 80206.

How we prepare the food we eat influences the quality of nourishment we obtain. Our emotional state while eating and digesting makes a difference also. Remember: eat only when hungry; not to fulfill or to cover up your feelings. Avoid eating when you're angry, tense, nervous, or in a hurry. At times like that, you're better off to just eat simple, easily digested foods. CHEW WELL. Food should disappear down your throat almost imperceptibly. If you have poor teeth, use a grinder or a juicer and then chew or swish the food around in your mouth so it will mix with the saliva. Stop eating when you feel satisfied; don't wait until you're stuffed. The principle of gradualness and moderation is important in making successful changes in food patterns. Change your diet thoughtfully. Use satisfaction as your guide. Experiment with recipes and keep successful ones.

GOOD FOOD COMBINATIONS

It makes sense to eat less meat, just from an ecological point of view: an average cow is given 21 pounds of protein to produce 1 pound of meat. This is an incredible waste. However, it's possible to raise your own animals more efficiently. A cow can eat grass and other humanly inedible roughage such as corn husks and pea vines, and convert this into meat. Animals that are raised at home, on land that has not been sprayed with chemicals, will produce very high quality milk and eggs and meat. Try to avoid store-bought meat. These animals have been shot up with antibiotics and artificial estrogens to hasten their growth. We consume some amount of these things when we eat such meat. The chickens are kept indoors without exercise, and their eggs have no taste, no substance, and they're barely yellow at all.

We can get excellent protein from non-meat sources by combining foods which have complementary amino acids. Frances Moore Lappe has done a thorough analysis of this process, which she explains in her book, Diet For a Small Planet

(Ballantine Books, 1971). The basic idea is that protein is **actually made up** of 22 amino acids. 8 of these are essential amino acids which **cannot be** synthesized by our bodies. At any given meal, all of these 8 essential amino acids must be present at the same time and in a particular proportion. If one or more of them is present in a disproportionately small amount, then your body will not be able to make use of the protein *as* protein, and that food will be used by the body for fuel, as if it were a carbohydrate. Seafood, dairy products, meat and poulty need no supplementation from other foods, but small amounts of these foods make excellent supplements in themselves. Wheat germ and eggs and rice are also good sources of whole proteins. Here are some guidelines for food combining for the optimal use of protein:

<u>SEAFOODS</u>: Cod and haddock are highest in protein. Combine seafood with Grains, Nuts, or Seeds. Example: fish and rice.

<u>DAIRY PRODUCTS</u>: These may be combined with Grains, Nuts, Seeds, Legumes, or Potatoes. Example: mashed potatoes with milk.

<u>LEGUMES</u> (dried peas, beans, lentils): Tofu (soybean curd) is even higher in protein than plain soybeans. Legumes should be eaten with Nuts, Seeds, or Grains, <u>and</u> Milk. Example: Peanut butter sandwich with milk.

<u>NUTS AND SEEDS</u>: Sunflower and sesame seeds are highest in protein. Sesame seeds are much more nutritious in their unhulled form, and far more digestible if ground. Cashews can be eaten alone as an excellent protein source. Nuts and Seeds are complemented by Legumes, Dairy Products, Seafood, <u>and</u> other Nuts and Seeds and Grains. Example: granola with milk.

<u>GRAINS, CEREALS</u>: Wheat, rye, and oats are highest in protein, especially hard red spring wheat and durum. Grains are complemented by Dairy Products, Legumes, Brewer's Yeast, and Nuts. Example: oatmeal with brewer's yeast.

TIPS FOR GOOD EATING

WHOLE GRAINS -- The best, most nutritious part of the grain is lost when you eat white flour, white rice, white cornmeal, or refined and instant-cooking cereals (rolled oats are okay). Most packaged cereals have the best part of the grains removed, and then nutrients are added artificially, along with lots of white sugar, artificial flavorings, and preservatives. 98% of the Vitamin E is lost in the process that makes cornflakes. 70% of the Vitamin E is lost in rice cereal products. So I recommend eating whole grains and whole grain products. You may want to get yourself a Corona Mill, so you can grind your own grains at home, for pancakes, cereal, and (if you're ambitious) bread. Grains begin to lose some of their nutrients within 2 hours after being ground, and a significant proportion is lost within 2 weeks. Also, corn begins to turn into carbohydrate 2 hours after it's picked, so this is an important vegetable to grow at home.

SALT -- Use Sea Salt, available in health food stores, because it's much higher in minerals than common table salt. Avoid canned and processed foods because they're highly oversalted.

SUGAR -- White sugar is the number one cause of tooth decay. The refining process concentrates the sugar to a degree where it can be harmful to the teeth, pancreas, and kidneys. Other sweeteners are preferable because they're less concentrated and contain beneficial minerals, but anything which is sweet and sticks to the teeth will cause tooth decay, so use all sweeteners in moderation. Dark raw honey, molasses, and maple syrup are all high in minerals. Brown sugar is better than white sugar simply because it contains molasses, which is an excellent nutrient.

BAKING POWDER -- Try to find a brand like Royal Cream of Tartar Baking Powder, which does not add aluminum.

CAFFEINE AND ALCOHOL -- Try to avoid or minimize these. They wash out your water soluble vitamins (B & C) and do other harm to your body.

The <u>I Ching</u> (an ancient Chinese book of wisdom) teaches us: Pay heed to the providing of nourishment and to what you fill your mouth with. What we take in and how we do it, strongly influences what we give out and the effect we have.

If you're nervous, there's probably a reason for it. You may know the reason and not be able to do anything to change it. Bioenergetic exercises are an excellent way of enabling the body to get rid of tension. Regular therapy may also be used to enable you to get at the root causes of your tension.

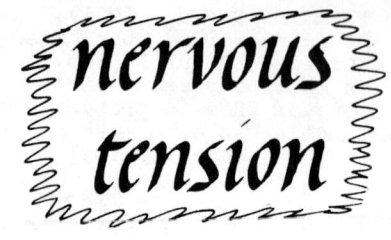

herbs

The following herbs may be used safely, to strengthen and feed the nerves while simultaneously easing nervous excitement, irritability, and pain.

1. VALERIAN, CATNIP, AND SCULLCAP: Bring 2 cups of water to a boil. Remove from heat. Add 1 tsp. each: valerian, catnip, and skullcap. Let sit for 20 minutes. Or take equal quantities of each herb (you can add hops and/or omit valerian, as you like) and grind in a coffee or other grinder (Molinex is good), and put in 00 gelatin capsules (available in some drugstores). Take as needed; 2-4 caps at a time or 1-2 cups of tea. If you want to sleep, you may need more. NOTE: some people are allergic to VALERIAN, and get stimulated instead of sedated, or get a stomach ache, dizziness, or nausea. Try in small quantities to begin with. If it does disturb you, then substitute hops instead.

2. HOPS: Boil 1 cup of water. Remove from heat. Add 1 tsp. hops. Let sit for 5 minutes. Drink as needed.

3. CALMS FORTE: A mild sedative, which is good for adults and safe for babies and small children (on special occasions like teething, long trips, or extreme pain). It contains plant extracts of passion flower, chamomile, oat, hops, and Biochemic Phosphates of Lime, Iron, Potash, Magnesia, and Sodium Chloride (Common Salt). These cell salts are in a form which permits ready assimilation and diffusion into the cells of the body. Calms Forte can be ordered from Standard Homeopathic Company, P.O. Box 61067, Los Angeles, Calif. 90061.

vitamin b

Frequently tension (stress) is caused or intensified by poor nutrition. B vitamins -- especially Niacin -- are important for your nerves. Try getting B vitamins regularly, in brewer's yeast or B Complex pills (Plus Products' Formula 72 is good). See also pages on Pregnancy for recipes for brewer's yeast. Also eat regularly, and plan balanced meals; see Centerfold for guidelines on Nutrition.

yoga

It's important to be able to relax. Often Yoga will be extremely helpful in achieving this end. There are good books that give excellent relaxing exercises and classes are taught at reasonable prices in most cities.

insomnia

Recent research on insomnia indicates that loss of sleep does no discernible harm to the body other than to make you feel sleepy. Sleeping pills interfere with your ability to dream. Some people benefit from vigorous outdoor exercise (like jogging) a few hours before bedtime. (Exercise just before bed will stimulate instead of relaxing.) If you can't get much sleep, it's probably better to get up and use your time constructively rather than try to force yourself to sleep. Also, it's a good idea to wait until you _feel_ sleepy, before you try to go to bed. Some people need less sleep than others; this is true for older people generally. Any of the remedies mentioned on this page may be used safely to help induce sleep. We particularly recommend the Valerian, Catnip, & Scullcap Tea (recipe above) -- one cup relaxes, and 2-3 cups make you sleepy. Sage Tea is also useful for Insomnia (cover 1 tsp. Sage with 1 cup boiling water and brew 5 minutes). If you have a lot of hops, you can make a HOPS PILLOW. Sprinkle the hops with a little alcohol, to activate their properties before using it as stuffing. This was a traditional Indian remedy for folks (especially children) who had trouble sleeping.

bladder infections

general advice

If you have trouble urinating, you may have a bladder infection but it's hard to diagnose. The symptoms -- burning urine, frequent urinating and pain in the bladder can be an indication of many things. The first is venereal disease. Men who get VD will almost always have these symptoms. If there is fever and backache accompanying the other symptoms, there is a chance of kidney disease. If the symptoms persist or come back again, especially the fever, it could be serious and you should see a doctor. Your kidneys are vital and shouldn't be messed with. However, in many cases you'll have a bladder infection, and there are things you can do about that. Women particularly get bladder infections often, due to the fact that their urethra is very close to their sex organs and they can be infected during intercourse.

If you think you have a bladder infection:

1. Get a urine test to make sure it isn't hep, VD, nephritis or some other serious disease.
2. Urinate before and after you make love, and after, drink 2-4 glasses of water. Urine is a good culture medium for bacteria to grow in, and pissing washes out whatever is in there.
3. For women, wipe yourself from front to back to avoid contaminating yourself with your own feces.
4. Rest a lot and cut down on strenuous work.

nutrition

1. Drink lots of liquids, but not black tea, coffee, or alcohol. CRANBERRY JUICE is excellent. Also, cranapple and apple. Drink 3 or 4 big glasses of juice a day.
2. As with other infections, take lots of VITAMIN C (it works by making the urine real acidic, so bacteria can't grow in it).
3. You may want to go on an ALL-FRUIT DIET for a while.
4. Take 200-600 units per day of VITAMIN E while the infection is active and for 2 weeks afterward, to prevent scarring.

herbs

1. BLADDER TEA: First, combine the following ingredients:
    - 1 Tablespoon yarrow flowers and leaves
    - 1 Tablespoon bearberry (uva ursi)
    - 1 Tablespoon corn silk
    - 1-1/2 teaspoons juniper berries

Then boil 3 cups of water and add 1 Tbsp. ECHINACEA ROOT - simmer 20 minutes and then pour over 1-1/2 tsps. of the above mixture. Cover and let steep for 15 minutes. Drink 1 cup a day for a week.

2. ALSO, on the first day, take:
    Two 00 caps of powdered golden seal root followed by 1/2 glass warm water <u>and</u>
    1000 mgs. of vitamin C before each meal.

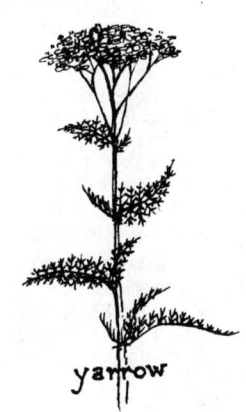
yarrow

women: vaginal infections

Cleanliness, diet, rest, and birth control methods are important factors in women's disorders. In Europe, women use bidets regularly. In America, you never see bidets, yet it's a very healthful practice for women (and men) to wash the genitals with clean clear water after intercourse (even if it's the next day). Soap of any kind should be avoided by women, because it interferes with the perfect acid-base balance of the vagina. Also, good diet, with plenty of B vitamins, and sufficient rest will help prevent vaginal infections. Hormone changes can often result in vaginal infections, which is why they so often occur during pregnancy, after menopause, and while taking birth control pills.

It's a good idea to learn how to examine yourself. You can see the first signs of a vaginal infection with a speculum exam before any itchiness or much discharge appears, and that's the best time to begin treatment. Some women's clinics and community clinics sell plastic speculums at cost (about 25¢) and will teach women how to use them. Self-examination also provides pregnancy detection, as you can notice the bluish change in your cervix as well as feel it softening.

The kind of symptoms that go with vaginitis -- discharge, itching, burning, increased sensitivity -- are similar to those seen with venereal diseases, so if there's any chance that you may have been exposed to VD, it's a good idea to have a culture taken, just to make sure. It's also important to mention that gonorrhea can be spread to the throat. Ask to have a throat culture taken if you may have been exposed. Cultures can be done at any clinic. If you're sure you don't have VD, here are some things you can do yourself, which will often get rid of an infection --

yeast infections

Yeast is found on the skin, in the bowels, and in the vagina. Common symptoms are itching, irritation, a red vagina, and a white cheesy discharge. It grows because of an imbalance in the bacterial flora of the vagina, which should be largely lactobacilli - the same bacteria that makes yogurt from milk! That's why yogurt helps to rebalance the flora.

Birth control pills are notorious for upsetting this balance. Women with recurring yeast infections may want to use a different method of birth control. Diabetics also have to be very careful because the yeast fungus will thrive on the excess sugar in their system. Yeast infections occasionally can be contracted by sexual contact so contact should be avoided during treatment. Broad-spectrum antibiotics like tetracycline and ampicillin and also Flagyl, which is used for treating Trichomonas, kill off all kinds of bacteria in the body, including the good ones like lactobacilli, thereby creating a favorable environment for an overgrowth of the yeast. So we advise women to eat 2 Tablespoons of plain yogurt 3 times a day and women who are very susceptible to yeast are advised to douche daily with yogurt (see below) while taking antibiotics. To treat yeast:

1. GARLIC SUPPOSITORIES: please see complete instructions on next page, under Trichomonas.
2. YOGURT: a vaginal applicator may be used to insert 2 Tablespoons of plain, natural yogurt (available from health food stores) into the vagina, twice a day, followed by a tampax OR a yogurt douche*may be prepared by using 4 Tablespoons of yogurt to 1 quart warm water, twice a day for 5 days or until the symptoms are gone, plus a few days.

*Douche: When douching, be careful not to force the infection up into the tubes: don't hang the bag more than 2 feet above the pelvis, and control the flow of water so that it enters very slowly.

women
page two

vaginal infections

trichomonas

Trich is caused by a tiny protozoa, a one-cell organism. Symptoms may be a yellow to yellowish-green discharge and a bad odor. Men are usually asymptomatic sometimes so are women. It can be passed during sexual contact (men can have it, not know it, and pass it on.) The usual treatment was Flagyl pills, but Flagyl has been found to cause cancer in animals, so most doctors have stopped using it. Trichofuron was considered a good substitute, but it was found to be so harmful that it was taken off the market. Now researchers in the <u>British Journal of Venereal Diseases</u> report that spermicidal jellies (like the kind used with diaphragms) inhibit the growth of trichomonas and yeast. <u>Liberation News Service</u> reports that some women who are very susceptible to trich infections (like many women who use birth control pills) have found that using spermicidal jelly every 2 weeks could prevent trich. Jelly can be inserted into the vagina with a foam applicator. Both the jelly and the applicator are available in most drugstores. (See also page 40 on Diaphragms and spermicidal jelly.)

<u>For WOMEN, we suggest</u>:
1. GARLIC SUPPOSITORIES: Prepare a garlic suppository by carefully peeling one small clove of garlic (don't nick the garlic, or it may burn) and placing it at the center of a piece of gauze, about 1 foot long and 3 or 4 inches wide. Fold the gauze in half and twist it around the garlic, making a kind of tampax with a gauze tail. Now dip the garlic end in vegetable oil, to make it easier to put in. Insert into the vagina. Change every 12 hours for 3-5 days.   OR ....
2. BETADINE: This is an antiseptic, available in most drugstores. Some clinics now use this instead of Flagyl. Put 1 Tbsp. Betadine in 1 pt. warm water and use as a douche, twice a day for 3 days and then once a day for 7 days (use less often if it's too irritating). Also, douche with yogurt on the 4th day and then every 2 days until the treatment is finished, to help avoid yeast infections (see pg. 36)

<u>For MEN</u>:
ABSTAIN for 10 days or use a condom -- then the organism can't survive. Follow this procedure for <u>everyone</u> you sleep with, or you will be rejuvenating the organism. Get checked again after 10 days, to make sure the Trichomonas is gone.

<u>GENERAL ADVICE</u>:
1. Get plenty of BED REST; trich may be caused by general exhaustion.
2. Maintain an ADEQUATE DIET, which would enable you to resist a parasitic infection. Get plenty of Vitamin A, the B Vitamins (Plus Products, Formula 71 is good), and protein.

bacterial infections (hemophilus, non specific) & cervicitis

Bacterial infections of the vagina are common, especially Hemophilus. These infections may cause a yellow, sometimes mucousy discharge, and some itching and/or irritation. There are other kinds of bacteria but they're usually not identified under the microscope so they're called "non-specific vaginitis." These are traditionally treated with triple sulfa vaginal cream (by prescription). The treatment below may be used for bacterial infections <u>and</u> CERVICITIS.

1. VINEGAR AND GARLIC: add 2 Tbsp. white vinegar (apple cider vinegar tends to ferment) and oil from 1 clove of garlic to 1 qt. warm water. Use as a douche, 2 times a day for 3-5 days (see footnote on douching, previous page). Garlic oil is available in some supermarkets, or cut 5 cloves garlic into fine pieces and cover with ½ cup plus 2 tbsp. vinegar and let sit all day. Then strain, and use 2 Tbsp. of this vinegar in your douche.   OR ....
2. GARLIC SUPPOSITORIES: see description above, under Trichomonas.

women
cramps
page three

iud — *intra uterine device*

Some cramping is to be expected, but if the pain becomes severe or your temperature goes up, get it checked out because it could be a sign of a pelvic inflammatory disease. Many women have found relief from cramps and discomfort by drinking the following teas, hot:

    MOTHERWORT and/or RASPBERRY LEAF: cover 2 tsps. of leaves with 2 cups of boiling water -- let brew for 5 minutes. Drink freely.

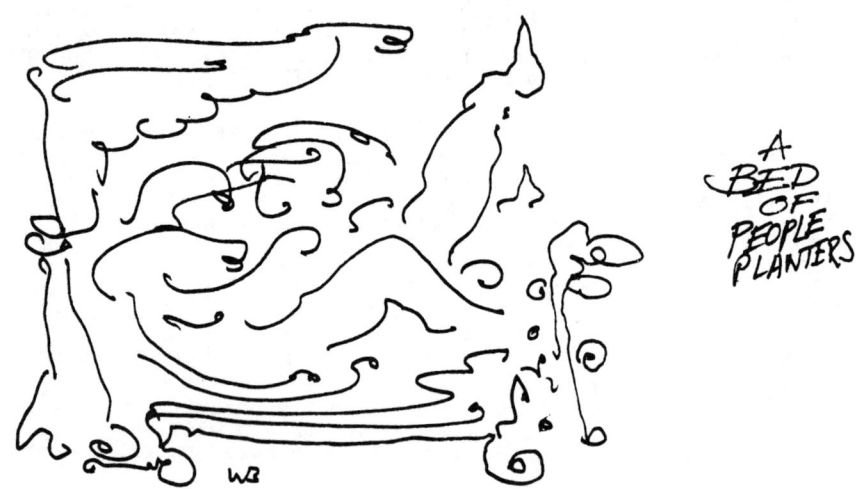

A BED OF PEOPLE PLANTERS

menstrual

1. CALCIUM: The level of calcium in the blood begins to drop about 10 days before the menstrual period begins, and for about 3 days after it begins. Calcium deficiency is characterized by: tension, nervousness, headaches, insomnia, mental depression, water retention, low resistance, and muscular cramps. To avoid menstrual difficulties, try increasing your calcium intake (see pages on Vitamins) as much as 10 days before your period is due. For cramping during your period, try taking a calcium pill every hour until the pain stops. Stop if diarrhea occurs.

2. HERBS: The following teas, which are also high in calcium, may be taken freely to relieve cramps:
    MOTHERWORT and/or RASPBERRY LEAF: see recipe above.
    COMFREY ROOT: boil 2 cups of water -- add 2 tsps. comfrey root -- simmer 20 minutes. Another herb, such as peppermint, may be added for flavor at the end. (i.e., remove from heat, add 2 tsps. peppermint, and brew 5 more minutes)

3. BIOFLAVANOIDS: Recent studies -- as shown in Prevention Magazine -- indicate that bioflavanoids help regulate the periods and prevent cramping. These can be bought as supplements in health food stores, or eaten in the whites and the pulp of organic citrus fruit (the skins of non-organic citrus are saturated with powerful insecticides) or in green peppers.

birth control

the ovulation method

There are so many factors which make coils, loops, and pills dangerous, unhealthful, and frightening, that I'd like to recommend yet another, and --some of us believe -- safer (when all factors are considered), method of birth control. This method enables you to reach an understanding of your own body and your own personal cycles, which are the tools you need in order to achieve or prevent pregnancy.

The Ovulation Method is based on the cervical mucous secretion: the normal vaginal discharge which changes according to the level of ovarian and pituitary hormones and thus indicates fertile and infertile days. This method was discovered by 2 Catholic doctors -- Drs. Lyn and John Billings -- out of dissatisfaction with the rhythm method. I've heard that it has now been recognized by the Pope.

The Ovulation Method has been studied by the World Health Organization, in their book, Cervical Mucus in Human Reproduction, which gives documentation of actual changes in the human body at the time of ovulation. Stated briefly: two kinds of secretions can be found in a healthy woman's vagina; the secretion produced in the vagina in response to sexual stimulation, and the cervical mucous which comes down from the cervix (the neck of the uterus). Just before ovulation, this cervical mucous has its own peculiar characteristics: it resembles egg white; it's very slippery, and can be "stretched" without breaking. To test this, when the mucous has a slippery quality, get some on the index finger, then touch the thumb to the mucous and slowly move the thumb away from the index finger. The mucous should stretch out in long strands between the two fingers. You don't need a speculum to examine the mucous; whatever is secreted by the cervix will come to the outside. You'll probably notice it when you wipe yourself after urinating. Then the finger can be inserted slightly into the vagina and the mucous can be observed. After observing the mucous closely for a full cycle between periods, you'll become aware of the changes it undergoes. You can learn to identify the ovulation mucous, and then, if your observation is correct, the menstrual period will begin 11-16 days after the ovulation mucous reaches its peak. Since semen closely resembles the consistency of ovulation mucous, instructors generally ask women to abstain for one month before using the method, in order to observe their mucous without confusion.

This technique of birth control is based on the following physiological observations: Estrogen, one of the female hormones, increases until it reaches its peak, at which time another hormone, luteinizing hormone, is released in the female body, causing an ovum to erupt from the ovary and to begin its journey down the fallopian tube, where it can be fertilized. At the same time, the rise in estrogen level causes the os (the mouth of the uterus, through which the sperm has to travel to reach the ovum) to open up. During this time, the Ovulation Mucous stretches itself into a corridor pattern which leads the sperm directly up to the uterus. And these corridors actually vibrate within the same frequency range as the tails of the sperm! And -- as if this wasn't enough -- the Ovulation Mucous is richly supplied with glucose, to nourish the welcomed sperm, so that it may live and fertilize for as long as $5\frac{1}{2}$ days.

This special Ovulation Mucous not only enhances the possibility of conception, it is necessary for it. After ovulation, the tacky, sticky cervical mucous sets in and the os closes up. Then the cervical mucous blocks the cervix and the relatively closed os with a cob-webby pattern of mucous which helps prevent the sperm from getting through. This kind of mucous is high in leucocytes (white blood cells) which surround the sperm and ingest them. It also contains anti-trypsin. Trypsin is the enzyme in the head of the sperm which enables the sperm to break down the outer shell of the egg and enter it.. Finally, this mucous also contains factors which tend to clump the sperm and stop the movement of their tails. Most sperm cannot survive more than a few hours in such an unfriendly medium.

* This section was written with the help of Nealy Gillette, author of The Ovulation Method: Cycles of Fertility.

birth control *page two* ovulation method (cont.)

The problem, then, is to learn to identify the ovulation mucous. This method works even if your periods are irregular, or you're coming off the pill, or if you've just had a baby, or before menopause when the periods are unpredictable. By observing the mucous each day, you can tell when you're ovulating, and by avoiding these days, you can avoid unwanted pregnancies. Or it can help you to conceive, if you deliberately have unprotected intercourse on your fertile days.

Some women prefer to abstain during the 7-14 days of possible fertility (it may be more days for women with very long cycles). This is the method recommended by Dr. John Billings in his book, <u>Natural Family Planning, The Ovulation Method</u>, available from The Liturgical Press, Collegeville, Minn. His book provides a simple explanation of the method, complete with calendars and stick-on labels, to mark your fertile days. Another excellent book which does not have a Catholic orientation is <u>The Ovulation Method: Cycles of Fertility</u> by Denise Guren and Nealy Gillette. It's available from Denise Guren, 4760 Aldrich Rd., Bellingham, Wa. 98225.

Since ovulation is generally a time of heightened sexual energy, abstinence may be undesirable. A diaphragm is a reasonably safe method of birth control to use during fertile and possibly-fertile days (see page 41). Withdrawal, or any direct contact between sexual organs is definitely not recommended on a fertile day, because pre-ejaculatory sperm is very fertile, and the ovulation mucous is easily penetrated.

IT IS NOT RECOMMENDED THAT ANYONE USE THE OVULATION METHOD WITHOUT INSTRUCTION. The mucous pattern is best taught by women who have used and understand the method from experience, and who can share a basic understnading of the physiological changes. Classes usually involve a 1½-2 hour presentation with follow-up about a month later. To obtain the names of teachers in your area, send a self-addressed, stamped envelope to The Ovulation Method Teacher's Association, P.O. Box 14511, Portland, Oregon 97214.

WARNING: The Ovulation Method has so far proved to be 95.5% effective for women who use it properly. But I have heard a few rare reports of women who became pregnant while using the method as taught. In each case, intercourse occurred during the <u>pre</u>-ovulatory phase. Dr. Val Donohue (Director of Gynecologic Oncology at Beth Israel Hospital in Boston, Massachusetts) says, "I believe that persistent survival of the sperm deep within the glands and clefts of the endocervical canal permits fertilization long after the original coitus .... Sperm can live happily in the alkaline pH of these glands for up to six days following intercourse." If this is possible, then it's safe to say that in order to have <u>maximum</u> protection against pregnancy, it is inadvisable to have unprotected intercourse until several days <u>after</u> ovulation has clearly occurred. The best rule of thumb is that when there is any doubt, use protection.

astrological birth control

In a previous edition of <u>Healing Yourself</u>, Astrological Birth Control was recommended. Since then, I've found that very few women felt comfortable with this concept of birth control. And only women with very regular cycles could use it safely. This method was developed by a Czechoslovakian doctor, Eugen Jonas, in the mid-fifties. Since the invasion of Czechoslovakia by Russia in 1968, Dr. Jonas has been out of touch with the rest of the world. Subsequent statistics and studies have been less favorable than those made by Jonas himself. Women following the Ovulation Method have had intercourse on the "astrologicaly fertile" days, and have not conceived. I now feel that the Ovulation Method is a technique which is more reliable than Astrological Birth Control. Some of the women who formerly taught ABC now teach only the mucous method.

birth control *page three*   the diaphragm

The diaphragm does not interfere with the body's hormones; it does not have any undesireable side-effects; it is almost as 'safe' as the pill or IUD and considerably safer than foam or rubbers. It is considered 98% reliable, when used with spermicide and used consistently and correctly. Some women prefer to just use a diaphragm all the time; other women enjoy knowing their own cycles, and use the diaphragm only during the period when there is a chance of impregnation (see pg. 39). The diaphragm does have the disadvantage of having to be inserted when you make love; on the other hand, it also has the very considerable advantage of being able to be removed. It allows your body to rest. It does not have to interfere with spontaneity entirely, because it's okay to insert the diaphragm as much as two hours before intercourse. Diaphragms have to be lubricated with either a jelly or a cream because this is what actually kills the sperm.

Instructions with the diaphragm say, every time intercourse is repeated within the 8 hour period after insertion, more spermicide should be injected without removing the diaphragm. And yet, in the August, 1975 iss.e of MS Magazine, Paula Weideger says, "These often annoying instructions do not seem grounded in the facts of spermicide life." She sites Dr. Hans Lehfeldt, Director of Family Planning at Bellevue Hospital in New York City whose studies have shown that spermicides remain active for 24 hours. The diaphragm still must remain in the vagina for 6 hours after the last intercourse, to be sure that no live sperm remain in the vaginal canal after the diaphragm is removed. But this still leaves 18 hours from the time the diaphragm is inserted, during which a woman should be protected by the same spermicide, no matter how many times intercourse takes place. Dr. Helena Wright, in her book, CONTRACEPTIVE TECHNIQUE, concurs with this opinion.

Paula Weidegger then points out that there are some disadvantages to be aware of in using the diaphragm: "Masters and Johnson...have found that the diaphragm may be displaced during intercourse, because the vaginal barrel expands during periods of sexual excitement. The danger of this happening is increased by repeated intercourse in the female-superior position. In such a situation the penis may be inadvertently inserted between the upper vaginal wall and the diaphragm. Sperm would then directly touch the cervix. Repeated intercourse in this position would then probably remove most of the spermicide left covering the cervix." For these reasons, we suggest the Ovulation Method, and refraining from actual intercourse during the few days when the vaginal mucous is stringy. The fertile days could be used to explore other methods of sexual gratification. Then the diaphragm could be used only on the days when there would be a slight chance of pregnancy. Or -- if this were undesireable -- at least the female-superior position and repeated intercourse could be avoided during periods of stringy mucous.

CREAM OR JELLY? You'll probably want to try both the cream and the jelly to decide which one you like the best. The cream is heavily perfumed, and many women prefer the smell and texture of the jelly, which they feel provides better lubrication. Some women have experienced signification irritation from Ortho brand jelly. There is a chemical irritant in Ortho which is not used in most other jellies, like Koromex or Ramses. But Koromex should be used with Koromex diaphragms, because it will discolor Ortho diaphragms. Koromex jelly used to have mercury in it, but they've discontinued the use of mercury.

TYPES OF DIAPHRAGMS: Before purchasing a diaphragm, don't be shy about handling it, testing the spring (in the circumference), feeling the texture of the rubber. Some springs are flat and very flexible (coil) and others are designed to bend only at a particular angle (arching spring). The latter are made for women whose cervix is deeper in the vagina, in order to give a tighter fit and therefore be safer. Also, some diaphagms are made of thick rubber and some of thin rubber. Community clinics or family planning centers will tend to be more cooperative than most pharmacists in letting you handle and examine the diaphragm.

HOLES -- CHANGE OF SIZE: It's a good idea to get a new diaphragm every year, to be sure it doesn't get a hole in it. If you don't use it often, you can wait 2 years. Check it yourself occasionally by holding it up to the light. After childbirth, or a miscarriage, or abortion, or a weight gain or loss of over 15 pounds, or if you were fitted before the hymen was broken, get the size checked again.

Pregnancy & child birth

From the time of conception and for a period of time after the delivery of the newborn infant, a pregnant woman becomes increasingly sensitive and susceptible to vibrations in her external and internal environments. A quiet, restful, yet open dwelling, pure air and water, plentiful wholesome food, and a little help from good friends provide the ultimate atmosphere for new human growth. It is hoped that the hints provided in this section will aid in achieving this goal.

precautions

Be extremely cautious about taking any amount of pharmaceutical, herbal, or psychedelic drugs during pregnancy. This applies especially to pills, capsules, rectal suppositories, or injected materials which bypass the body's chemical monitors (senses of taste and smell). Most women find that their senses are very finely tuned when they're pregnant, and they get very definite messages about what they should and shouldn't eat. Believe in your senses -- they're usually your best advisors.

Preferred treatment forms are oral solutions (teas, drops, etc.), and topical applications for local therapy (eye and ear preparations, non-absorbable vaginal medications, skin creams, etc.).

From the 15th day after conception (about the time the first missed period is due) until the end of the third month of pregnancy, the fetus is undergoing the very delicate task of forming all its organs. Exposure to drugs or toxic agents during this time should be strictly avoided. Even massage should not be too rough. Acupuncture should be done only by a master.

a few specifics to avoid

MSG MONOSODIUM GLUTAMATE (ACCENT): This very common food additive gives a meat-like or sometimes sweet flavor to foods - and causes brain damage to experimental infant animals when given in large amounts. MSG is found in many canned foods (soups, vegetables, etc.), and is used extensively in restaurant cooking (especially oriental cooking). It is also present in soy sauces either as a chemical additive (Kikkoman) or as a product of natural fermentation (Tamari). The natural product is less harmful and should be insisted upon, yet not indulged in to obvious excess.

GOLDEN SEAL (HYDRASTIS): Golden Seal has been used for centuries as a cardiac stimulant and uterine contractant. As it is known to produce expulsion of the fetus in certain pregnant animals, it should be used cautiously during pregnancy, if at all. Two or three "00" capsules of Golden Seal powder contain a dose of Hydrastine (one of the effective ingredients of the herb) large enough to start a premature labor. Take care with this herb.

KITTY LITTER BOX: Cats are frequent carriers of the protozoa which causes Toxoplasmosis. These organisms are constantly shed into the cat's shit where they become infectious to people after several days' incubation. Toxoplasmosis is characterized by the same symptoms as a common cold in adults. If a woman has toxo once, then she is immune to it. But if a pregnant woman with no immunity to toxoplasmosis is exposed to these organisms, the result may be infection of the fetus causing extensive brain damage. Unfortunately, there is no convenient test to check a person's immunity to Toxo, so prevention rests on reducing exposure to cat feces as much as possible. If a pregnant woman has cats around, it is best if a non-pregnant friend empties the cat box frequently. Toxoplasmosis in newborn people is a rare disease -- let's make it even more rare.

CIGARETTES: Cigarettes release toxins in the body which reduce the amount of oxygen that reaches the cells. Then the body has to use energy -- which would otherwise be available for growth (the baby) and repair - to break down those toxins. Every cigarette you smoke destroys 20 mg's of Vitamin C in your body. Try to at least reduce your cigarette intake by half and get plenty of Vitamin C.

A PARTIAL LIST OF KNOWN TOXIC AGENTS, DRUGS, AND HERBS: aspirin, blue cohash, cat feces, ergot and derivatives (LSD), golden seal, mistletoe, MSG (Accent), pennyroyal, flagyl (Metranidazole), paint and solvent fumes, sulfa drugs (during 9th month), tansy, tetracycline, common tobacco, Vitamin C (over 5 grams/day), Vitamin E in massive doses, Western red cedar, wild celery root (osha)

pregnancy & child birth   page two

what you should eat

Perhaps the most important factor in assuring a normal pregnancy and a healthy newborn child is good nutrition. If possible, this should start before conception so that the mother has some reserves. Although food can be used as therapy for difficulties which may arise during pregnancy (anemia, etc.), it is much better to prevent these complications before they occur by eating properly throughout the pregnancy.

The best assurance of getting the proper amounts of proteins, minerals, and vitamins is to eat a good variety of whole, fresh foods. Emphasis should be placed on lean meats, whole grains, milk, cheese and eggs supplemented by fresh green and yellow vegetables, fruits (both citrus and other), potatoes with skins, unrefined vegetable oils, nuts and seeds, and - of course - natural flavorings. Please see pages 32-33 on PROVIDING NOURISHMENT.

A pregnant woman should eat enough to satisfy her appetite. A weight gain of 20 to 40 pounds during the 9 months can be expected. Most of this is usually lost after birth, especially if the baby is breast-fed, but if one gains as much as 40 pounds, it may be difficult to lose later.

Getting enough of the proper foods may become difficult as the baby grows and presses on the stomach, making it hard to eat large meals. In this case nutritious, ready-to-eat snacks should be made available around the clock to insure good food intake. Do not rely on preservative-laced foods, which may do more harm than good. Fresh roasted nuts, refrigerated cuts of cooked meat, cheese slices, a salad with dressing ready, bread with jam and butter, natural peanut butter and jelly sandwiches on whole grain bread with milk, fresh fruit, etc. should be stocked in ample supply.

The following recipes are easy to prepare, satisfying, and excellent sources of iron, protein, and B and C vitamins. Ingredients for these should be on hand at all times:

TIGRESS' MILK

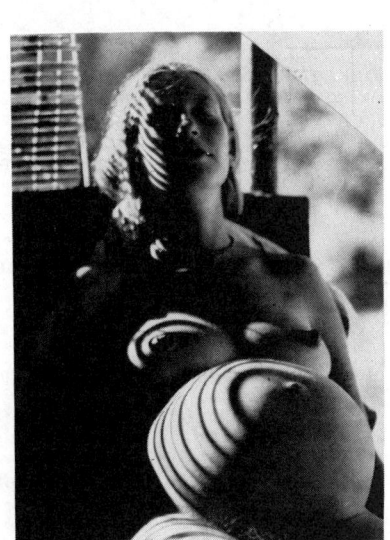

1/4 cup to 1 cup whole milk (depending on desired consistency)
1/4 cup yogurt
Juice of one orange OR
1/4 cup frozen orange juice concentrate
1 1/2 Tbsp. Torula or Brewer's Yeast
1 Tbsp. blackstrap molasses
1 Tbsp. wheat germ
1/4 Tsp. vanilla extract
Dash of nutmeg

Stir this all together or blend in a blender and drink it down. Fantastic!

YOGURT DELIGHT

Fill a bowl with plain YOGURT. Add Torula or Brewer's YEAST to taste (as much as possible). Plenty of WHEAT GERM comes next, then a tablespoon of BLACKSTRAP MOLASSES. Finally add pieces of dried or fresh FRUIT (raisins, apricots, strawberries, bananas, etc.) Top with frozen orange juice or pineapple-orange juice concentrate if desired. Stir and eat.

pregnancy and child birth
page three
important nutrients

protein

A pregnant or nursing woman needs a lot of protein. Doctors and midwives often suggest 85-100 grams a day, but many vegetarian women get less and do very well. The Required Daily Allowance for nonpregnant women is about 45; during pregnancy it goes up to 75; and during lactation it's 65.

Dr. Tom Brewer advises pregnant women to eat a daily diet of at least 1 quart milk or yogurt, 2 eggs, and 2 servings of fish, poultry, meat, cheese, or combinations of non-meat foods to make whole proteins.

Foods that contain about 15 grams of protein include: almonds (½ cup), cashew nuts (1 cup), peanuts (1/3 cup), cheese (2½ oz.), eggs (2), full-fat soy flour (1/3 cup), whole wheat flour (1 cup), cooked beans (1 cup) including lentils, split peas, soybeans, lima beans, and red kidney beans; crab, lobster, and shrimp (3½ oz.); fish, turkey, chicken, beef, and bacon (2 oz.).

If you don't eat meat, it's useful to know how to combine food groups to get all the amino acids necessary to make up full proteins. This is explained in DIET FOR A SMALL PLANET by Frances Moore Lappe. One simple rule-of-thumb in planning meals or snacks is to divide foods into the following 4 groups, and then choose combinations from at least 2 groups:
1 - grains; 2 - beans; 3 - nuts and seeds; 4 - dairy

For example, a peanut butter sandwich combines nuts (the peanut butter) and grains (the bread). A multi-grain bread will probably contain grains (such as wheat) and beans (such as soy flour) or seeds (like flaxseed). A cheese taco combines dairy (cheese) and grains (corn tortilla).

fats & oils

Little attention is given to these nutrients, yet they are absolutely essential for human growth. Butter and vegetable oils are the best sources. Safflower, peanut, olive, and soy oils are all very suitable. Hain's makes an All-Blend oil which is excellent. Other sources are avocados, real mayonnaise, peanuts and non-hydrogenated peanut butter. Look for naturally cold-pressed oils, and avoid preservatives such as BHA and BHT. 2 Tablespoons of oil per day, used in cooking or salads, is ample.

iron

Iron is one of the most difficult minerals to obtain in quantity from food. About 1/3 of the mother's iron supply is taken by the baby to form its blood. During pregnancy, your blood supply will increase from ¼ to ½ the amount you had before pregnancy. This shouldn't cause any problem as long as you eat well, and have no trouble with bleeding -- which is the only way your body can lose a lot of iron. Iron losses are replaced very slowly, so if there has been a problem before pregnancy with anemia or heavy menstrual bleeding or other blood loss, have the blood count checked.

The hematocrit is a blood test which indicates the number of red cells in the blood. It's taken by pricking the finger for blood. Red cells carry iron, so a low count may indicate iron deficiency anemia. The red cells are also vital because they carry oxygen to the baby's body, and your own. (Please see page 58 for best food sources of Iron.)

calcium

The RDA for an adult woman is 800, but while pregnant and nursing, it jumps to 1200. If you don't get enough calcium, your baby will get it from your teeth and bones (via the blood), leaving your body weaker and more susceptible to problems like osteoporosis in later life. If you're not getting enough calcium, you may be having problems such as leg cramps (Charlie Horse), spasms, and greater susceptibility to pain. (Please see page 57 for best food sources of Calcium.)

pregnancy & child birth — page four

vitamin a

Vitamin A is necessary for proper development and upkeep of the eyes and skin. While pregnant and nursing, you need about twice as much as other adults. (Please see page 53 for best food sources.)

b vitamins

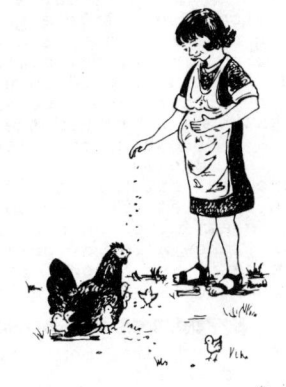

The 12 different substances which compose the B Complex form the basis for all cellular growth and multiplication. Lack of the B's can cause anemias, nerve and mental disorders, diarrhea, skin difficulties, and lack of appetite to the point of weight loss. Obviously, the B's are extremely important during pregnancy. By far the best source of this vitamin is brewer's type yeast. Donsbach Yeast 500 is especially good because of its high folic acid content.

Folic acid is one of the B vitamins, and it's particularly important during pregnancy because a deficiency of this nutrient can cause pregnancy mask or toxemia. You should be getting about 800 mcg. per day.

Vitamin B6 (pyridoxine) is also vital during pregnancy, and one source says that 95% of all pregnant women are deficient. Symptoms include nausea and vomiting, leg cramps, nervousness, irritability, lack of energy, insomnia, bad-smelling gas, hemorrhoids, and anemia. Vitamin B should always be taken as a whole complex. See page 54.

vitamin c

This multi-purpose vitamin is necessary for the production of tissue proteins which hold us and our babies together. Note: Doses over 5 grams per day may be dangerous during the first trimester. See page 56.

vitamin d

Vitamin D is necessary for calcium utilization and bone formation. Deficiency in infants causes the bowed legs of rickets. See page 56.

vitamin e

Vitamin E is essential for prevention of habitual miscarriage. It also protects against asphyxiation due to insufficient oxygen -- a factor of considerable importance to the baby during labor. Vitamin E oil is often beneficial in preventing and/or reducing the appearance of scars and stretch marks when applied to the skin daily for long periods.

vitamin k

Vitamin K is essential for proper blood coagulation. Deficiencies of K cause excessive bruising or bleeding from minor injuries. Good sources of K are found in all dark green leafy vegetables (kale, cabbage, spinach, etc.), tomatoes, and alfalfa (which may be taken as sprouts or tablets, but not as tea because this vitamin is not water-soluble). The bacteria in the human gut also synthesize a lot of K, but these bacteria are destroyed by taking sulfa or antibiotic drugs, in which case additional dietary intake of this vitamin is strongly advised. Additional K is also recommended if a woman becomes jaundiced during pregnancy, as vitamin K absorption is decreased greatly in states of jaundice. Be sure to correct deficiencies before labor, to prevent dangerous hemorrhaging.

preparing for childbirth
limbering the body

pregnancy & childbirth   page five

Next to eating properly, keeping one's body in trim by good exercise is most important during pregnancy. Such exercise should never be harsh or carried to the point of physical exhaustion. Walking in pleasant surroundings is probably best. Swimming is also good. It's a good idea to get outdoors as much as possible, and wear loose, comfortable clothing that allows free movement. Most Yoga positions and postures are excellent for keeping limber, but avoid postures which place excess strain on the spine. Vaginal tightening and relaxing should be practiced before and after delivery. A good way to learn this exercise is to tighten one's pelvic floor muscles so as to stop the flow while urinating. Abdominal tightening will help the belly muscles to regain proper size and strength after the birth.

Breathing exercises are particularly important, especially in prepartion for natural birth. Breathing is the key to body-mind relaxation, thus its importance in labor and other stressful situations. The techniques for controlled breathing are many and varied.(Please see the list of Books on pregnancy and birth on page 64.) The importance lies in focusing one's attention on breathing - and only breathing. The rest of the body remains fully relaxed. This takes a lot of practice, so the sooner a suitable technique is learned, the better. Seeing if the discomfort of a "horsebite" applied to one's knee can be overridden with breathing control is a convenient test of one's competence.

preparing the mind

Read all you can about pregnancy, childbirth, and newborn babies. Get as many different viewpoints as possible. Movies are good for birth preparation, but not as good as actually seeing a baby born. Talk to recent mothers about their experiences, and don't forget to ask older women what it used to be like. Remember, however, that no two births are ever alike, and that those with bad experiences often speak the loudest.

self-examination

It is possible for a woman, and her close friends if she wishes, to follow most of her physical changes during pregnancy, birth, and after. Some highlights are noted here.

The enlarging uterus can first be felt by pressing in on the belly above the pubic bone at 3 months. Breast tenderness and enlargement may be noticed at or before this time. At five months exactly, the top of the uterus is felt just at the bellybutton. Somewhat after this the baby's heartbeat can be heard using a good stethoscope. Friends can hear it by placing an ear on the belly. Take time in quiet surroundings to listen properly, and listen all over the uterus. By seven months the baby's parts can be felt. With time, practice, and good relaxation the head, back, buttocks, and legs become discernable. Around the eighth month the head should be located down near the pubic bone. The head can then be felt by vaginal self examination - done, of course with clean hands, well trimmed nails, and much gentleness. At first the head will be felt to be "floating". Later it becomes less moveable as it descends into the pelvis before labor. The cervical opening itself is located deep behind the head, and is usually difficult to reach. Never put a finger through the cervical opening, as premature breaking of the waters or infection could result.

Vaginal examination during labor is not advised between the time the waters first break until the baby can be seen between the vaginal lips. This precaution is also to prevent infection. As the baby's head crowns, however, it is very rewarding for the mother to reach down and touch it. In instances of exceptional control, it is even possible for the woman to deliver the baby from (to?) herself.

Immediately after the birth, as soon as the baby is breathing well, it can be placed on the mother's chest if the umbilical cord is long enough. The uterus should be felt about bellybutton level. Deep lower abdominal massage will contract the uterus if it cannot be felt; this helps stop bleeding. Nursing the baby on the breast also contracts the uterus. As the placenta is delivered, the uterus becomes a bit smaller, but should remain about the size and consistency of a grapefruit. Don't forget to look at the placenta, membranes, and cord. They are amazing structures, almost as interesting as the baby. The placenta should have no torn blood vessels running off its edge. If it does, the missing placental piece should be found.

Inspection for vaginal tears should be made after the birth. If these are deep, they should be sutured within 8 hours. A few days after delivery the vaginal lips can be self examined, perhaps with the aid of a hand mirror. Effectiveness of pelvic tightening exercises can be seen during these examinations.

As the milk comes in more and more, replacing the thin colostrum, the uterus becomes smaller and smaller, until in several weeks it can no longer be felt.

problems & some solutions — pregnancy & child birth

headaches
Aspirin is not recommended during the first three months of pregnancy as it may cause birth defects. Please see page 5 on Headaches.

Decay can occur very quickly, as can gum difficulties. Calcium deficiency may cause tooth problems. Please see page 13 on Teeth.

nausea - morning sickness
These problems are very common early in pregnancy, but are usually short lasting. Persistence of these symptoms may suggest that one's headspace and especially one's fears need to be worked through and understood. Many times the problem can be overcome simply by having something to eat immediately upon awakening. Crackers, bread, or toast placed at the bedside at night is a good remedy. Hot drinks such as milk or tea in a bedside thermos are also effective. Vitamins are particularly important at this time. Please see pages 54-55 on the B Vitamins. Page 9 on Nausea and Vomiting contains good remedies, most of which may be used during pregnancy. If the problem persists to the point of weight loss, be sure to consult a physician.

anemia
The blood count falls normally during pregnancy, but it should never be allowed to drop too low. If it does, be sure that blood loss is not the reason (Excessive menses before conception, bleeding during pregnancy, or bleeding into the gut causing black shit). Usually iron deficiency is at fault, but sometimes lack of B Vitamins (Folic acid and B-12) can cause anemia. Moderate anemia itself is not dangerous, and may even go unnoticed, but it leaves no reserve should there be excessive bleeding during the childbirth. Anemia tests (hematocrit) should be done at least at the beginning of pregnancy and during the seventh month, as it takes 2-3 months to build up the blood if necessary.

Anemia is best prevented by a diet with much protein, vitamins and iron. Please see page 57 for the best food sources of Iron. However if enough iron is still not present in the diet, a supplement of 15 mg. per day throughout pregnancy is advised. Strong cravings for odd foods may be the first sign that more iron is needed.

If iron therapy is necessary for a discovered anemia, it is suggested that Ferrous Fumarate, Gluconate, or Lactate be taken - not Ferrous Sulfate or Chloride, which are very harsh on the baby. Dosage is 100 mg. once a day for moderate anemia (hematocrit under 33%) or three times a day for dangerous anemia (under 30%). These dosages cause one's shit to become black. If supplements are taken, they should be followed 12 hours later by 100 I.U. of Vitamin E.

edema - toxemia
Edema is a term used for excessive fluid retention. This is characterized by swelling of the feet and ankles. Simple edema is usually relieved by keeping off your feet for a day or two. Lying down when resting, with the feet and hands raised above the level of the heart, relieves swelling by gravity. Try to avoid lying on your back because the uterus presses on the large vein, the vena cava, and restricts the blood flow from the legs. Lying on the left side gives the best blood return.

Edema in the last 6 weeks of pregnancy is a healthy phenomena, if there is no toxemia, and if there is proper nourishment. Edema is nothing to worry about by itself, however it is just symptom in a syndrome called toxemia, which is characterized by edema, high blood pressure, and protein in the urine.

Restriction of salt is not particularly helpful in relieving swelling, and may even be harmful by producing sodium deficiency. Sea salt -- not common salt -- is recommended because it is milder and contains more minerals than regular salt. Diuretics should not be taken during pregnancy.

VITAMIN B6: This vitamin is very effective in eliminating water retention. Doctors prescribe it routinely for the edema of pregnancy. We suggest 25-50 mg. per day. See page 54 for more information on taking specific B vitamins.

frequent urination
As the uterus grows and presses on the bladder, one must urinate more and more often - sometimes as much as every hour. Due to the anatomy involved, not much can be done about this problem. If there is pain on urinating, or if a fresh warm urine sample is cloudy (pee into a clear glass to check it), it is wise to have the urine examined microscopically to be sure a urinary infection is not also at fault. A urinal and toilet paper by the bedside will prevent toes being stubbed in the dark.

pregnancy & childbirth problems (cont.)
page seven

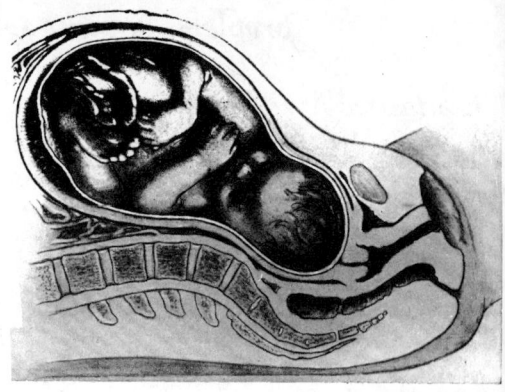

leg cramps

Sudden calf cramps are not uncommon during pregnancy. Low calcium levels may be a cause. Please see page 58 on Calcium for the best food sources, and a good supplement. A gram or two of calcium supplement daily should bring relief from further attacks. In a previous edition, we suggested quinine water, but we've since learned that quinine is contraindicated in pregnancy. (Even doctors make mistakes -- it was a doctor who originally suggested the quinine water.) To stop a cramp when it's happening, pull the toes and ball of the foot up towards the kneecap. If the calf is painful constantly, have the condition checked to make sure that phlebitis (vein inflammation) is not the cause.

vaginitis

The vast hormonal and chemical changes during pregnancy can cause overgrowth of otherwise friendly organisms living in the vagina. This produces a whitish discharge which may be quite annoying. It is best to have an exam to determine which bug is at fault - especially as gonorrhea is sometimes the cause. Vaginal infections are all hard to get rid of until after the birth. Therapy is aimed at suppressing the annoying symptoms.

Douching is just about as effective to this end as antibiotic therapy, and can be safely done in moderation up to the time the waters break <u>provided</u> that it is done gently and the vagina is allowed to drain freely (do not hold the labia together to fill the vagina by pressure). Small amounts of vinegar or yogurt added to warm water make effective and convenient douche preparations.

Suppositories, either herbal or prescription, must likewise be used with caution. Be certain to remove them after 24 hours if they do not dissolve. Flagyl tablets or suppositories should not be used during pregnancy.

Using a condom during intercourse, by keeping sperm out of the vagina, may decrease an otherwise bad discharge. See also pages 36-37 on Women: Vaginal Infections.

varicose veins

The hormonal changes during pregnancy cause the veins throughout the body to become more lax, thus predisposing to varicose veins. To make matters worse the weight of the uterus rests on the veins which drain the legs when standing or sitting. This increases the pressure in the leg veins, making them bulge even more.

Walking and exercising as much as possible, with avoidance of sitting for long periods provides the best prevention. Adelle Davis recommended kicking a pillow - hard, thus relieving tension and getting leg exercise at the same time. Vitamin B in moderate dosage may help veins which are already beginning to enlarge, to return to normal size. Please see pages 54-55 on the B vitamins.

Elevation of the legs is beneficial in collapsing the veins, thus giving them a rest. Likewise, placing the chest lower than the hips (such as getting on elbows and knees) brings the uterus up and out of the pelvis, allowing the leg veins better drainage. Properly fitted support stockings (Jobst) are useful if varicose veins are a problem. Stockings should be most snug toward the feet, so that the blood is squeezed up and out, and not trapped by tight bands or clothing.

hemorrhoids

Hemorrhoids are varicose veins occurring around the anus. The basic rules for treating leg varicose veins applies to hemorrhoids also. Pelvic tightening exercises are helpful in contracting the anus and pumping the blood out of enlarged pelvic veins. Virtually every woman has large hemorrhoids during labor due to the pressures involved. These disappear soon after giving birth, with the help of exercise. (See pg. 20, Hemorrhoids.)

herbal preparations to aid pregnancy

RED RASPBERRY LEAF TEA: Pour one cup boiling water over one tsp. dried leaves. Steep 3-5 minutes. May be sweetened or mixed with other teas such as peppermint. Said to prevent miscarriage and ease and shorten labor, besides being nutritious in itself and pleasant tasting Dose is one cup per day throughout pregnancy or 3 cups per day during the last 6 weeks.

SARSAPARILLA may be taken in the form of tea or the root may be chewed. It prepares the uterus for childbirth, helps prevent miscarriages, and eases the uterine spasms which sometimes follow birth. When buying Sarsaparilla, chew a little. If it doesn't have an acrid taste, it's no good. For tea, simmer 1 tsp. of root in 1 cup water for 20 minutes.

pregnancy & childbirth
(home & other deliveries)
page eight

Labor begins at the onset of rhythmic uterine contractions and ends with the completed separation of mother from child, plus placenta. During this time, the mother opens up, in both the physical and psychic sense of the word. She becomes increasingly sensitive to surrounding people and atmosphere so that a positive environment helps provide the fortitude and relaxation necessary for a quick and relatively easy birth. A negative, fear and anxiety producing atmosphere, however, can slow or even stop labor, thus requiring medical intervention.

Therefore, the pregnant woman must have the freedom to choose the medical consultant for the birth, as well as the other people to be present, and the place for the delivery. In selecting a medical consultant, it's wise to choose an experienced person who's guided at least twenty births, and is well versed in artificial resuscitation of the newborn, and in uterine massage (in case of hemorrhage). It is wise to make prior arrangements with a licensed physician, should complications arise. Having trust in the skill and judgment of one's consultant is of utmost importance for the generation of confidence.

The other people present should also be chosen to provide or reflect confidence. It should be borne in mind that labor is an incredible exposure and, for some, it is often highly sexually charged. Thus helpers who are comfortable with their own and others' bodies should be sought. Whether they be trained delivery assistants or one's friends, their job is to provide mental and physical support. The place of birth is likewise important. Whether it be a large hospital, a smaller birth clinic (these are unfortunately rare in the U.S.), one's home, or outdoors, the proper vibrations must be present for the most favorable outcome. If the setting is not optimum, the laboring woman should feel free to communicate to her helpers that a change is needed.

In American hospitals at present, anaesthetics, delivery forceps, and even Caesarian Section are much over-used. Each carries a definite risk to the baby and mother. Also the practice of inducing labor with Pitocin just so the birth can be scheduled for a certain day, subjects the baby to the risks of prematurity and a confused astrological sense. Labor and delivery are natural occurrences and will, in the vast majority, proceed without difficulty, especially if the mother is healthy, is trained in how to relax fully and breathe with the contractions, and the baby is facing head down (Vertex). To interfere with a natural process with harsh procedures and drugs is to invite danger.

In many institions today it is the practice as soon as the baby is born to immediately clamp the umbilical cord (thus depriving the baby of 20% of its blood which is still in the placenta) and hand the child to an assistant who rubs its skin harshly, suctions its throat and stomach, inspects it, injects it and then (after maybe a brief exposure to the mother) takes it down the hall to the nursery.

Many simpler societies consider this barbaric. The newborn infant is awake for about the first hour after birth, and it is during this time that it "imprints" most heavily on all its surroundings. After the child is delivered, be sure it is breathing. There is no need to spank the baby. If it's not breathing, just blow air on its navel, and this will usually cause it to gasp and start breathing. Or flick the soles of the feet. Now the blood is still flowing from the placenta into the baby, and you want to make the most of this "placental transfusion," so place the infant at a level below the placenta, and cover it with a receiving blanket or a soft cloth to prevent heat loss. The veings and arteries in the cord begin to collapse after a few minutes; wait until the cord is done pulsating and collapses before tying it.

labor brings

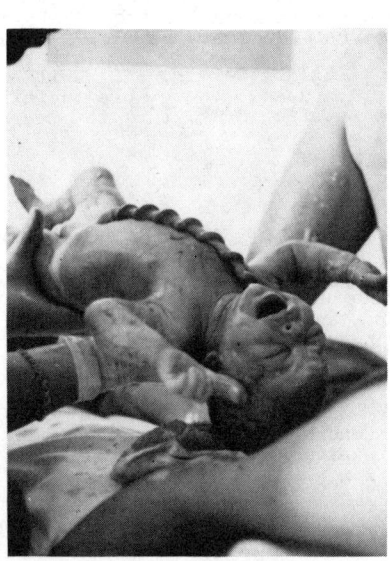

deliverance

home & other deliveries (cont.)

A friend can then take the baby gently and with a piece of cotton and wheat germ oil, the child can be cleaned and inspected and then returned to its mother. A soft blanket may be placed over the two of them to keep them warm. If the baby wishes to suckle, let it take the breast; this stimulation helps the uterus to contract. For the next hour, at least, let the mother and child and friends become acquainted by touching and close contact. Then the mother is assured of the reality of her experience and that the child is alive and well. And the child may feel and perhaps taste the warmth of its mother, and hear her familiar heart beat. It can recover from its long journey and sudden emergence onto dry land, and the light of day -- after being so long in that watery darkness.

Comfort your little one, and wait for the placenta. As much as half an hour may pass before the contractions come strong enough to deliver the placenta. Once it is delivered, inspect it to make sure there are no severed vessels running off the edge of it. Make sure it is whole. The placenta may then be disposed of by burying it or composting it. It also makes an excellent dish when sauteed with onions and herbs if the cord and membranes are first removed. It tastes like transcendental organic liver, and -- as every other animal knows -- it is the perfect nourishment for the new mother.

After delivery is complete, use a kotex pad. If six pads soon become soaked to the saturation point, it is a sign of danger. If help cannot be had, oral fluid replacement can be lifesaving. Give one teaspoon salt in 1 quart of water.

NOURISHMENT DURING LABOR

From the time that contractions begin in earnest until the mother's condition is once again stable after the birth, taking of solid foods or medicines should be avoided. This is to prevent vomiting, which could be dangerous should a labor become overwhelming or should anaesthetics be needed. In an emergency, if anaesthetics have to be used, one of the greatest dangers is that vomiting could occur and go into the lungs. Liquids in moderation may be taken slowly in sips. Fresh water can be very refreshing. Ice chips (perhaps made from mint tea with honey), hot tea, juices, or a hearty broth provide a good spectrum of nourishment.

GINGER TEA: Place 1 tsp. grated fresh ginger or 2 tsp. dried ginger pieces in 2 C. boiling water. Simmer 5 min. Drink hot. Strengthens spirits. Natural stimulant.

BRANDY: Alcohol should not be forgotten as an aid in labor. In moderate amounts (1/2 to 1 oz. brandy or whiskey) it aids relaxation of the pelvis and free passage for the baby. In larger amounts (4 oz. or so) it may slow or stop labor should an emergency arise (such as the cord coming first) so that help can be reached. If it tends to make you groggy or sleepy, we don't recommend it for normal labor.

VALERIAN, CATNIP, AND SCULLCAP TEA: If labor is prolonged and the muscles are tense, it is often useful to be able to fall asleep, to relax and re-gather strength. Instead of using a powerful drug, this tea may be prepared. Please see page 34 on Nervous Tension for recipe.

TO PREVENT OR STOP HEMORRHAGING

1. UTERINE MASSAGE: This should be used together with one of the following:

2. SHEPHERD'S PURSE TEA: This tea can be made during transition, to have ready after the birth. Use at least 1 heaping teaspoon per cup, and pour boiling water over the tea. Brew 3 minutes. Make it stronger if the situation predisposes to hemorrhage: if the labor is long, or if there is anemia or a history of previous hemorrhaging. Take as much as 3 cups right after the delivery of the placenta.

3. CAYENNE: Take two 00 caps (1/4 tsp.) of cayenne. If you don't have caps, take 1/4 tsp. of cayenne on the tip of a butter knife and put it at the back of your throat (where you don't have too many taste buds), then swallow down with warm water. Repeat. After about 10 minutes, this can be repeated again.

SEE A DOCTOR IMMEDIATELY IF THE BLEEDING DOES NOT STOP OR SIGNIFICANTLY LESSEN AFTER 15 MINUTES.

NOTE: This is obviously not a complete guide on home deliveries. Plese see page 64 for a list of books related to Pregnancy, Childbirth, Nursing, and Babies.

post-natal care   *pregnancy & childbirth*   page ten

you:

THE PERINEUM: If the perineum does tear in labor, it will be very sensitive for the next week or two. You can use a piece of cotton dipped in warm water and hold it on the perineum while urinating to help alleviate the stinging. The rest of the time the lochia (mucousy red flow) coats and soothes the tissues.

REST: Try to keep off you feet and let your body heal itself those first few days; don't be too anxious to prove how strong you are. If the blood flow picks up suddenly, slow down; you're doing too much. Don't forget to continue to eat well. And get plenty of rest. If you can take naps or go to bed early, it makes it a lot easier to wake up in the middle of the night with the baby. Especially during the first three months, try to arrange your life so that you (and hopefully the father and/or friends of the baby) will have plenty of time to be with the little one and give him or her lots of love and attention. On days when your energy level is low, don't force yourself to work if you don't have to. Save your high-energy days for work. Let your house get messy; let the baby come first for awhile. The first months with this new person are very special. Try to give yourself time to enjoy them.

DIET: Remember that your dietary requirements are even <u>higher</u> now, if you're nursing, than they were when you were pregnant. Please see preceeding pages. This is not the time to get anxious about getting slender. Do exercises to make yourself firm, but be tolerant about a little extra weight until the baby gets weaned.

the baby:

THE CORD: In hospitals, a chemical is painted on the cord to keep out organisms. But these organisms are harmless, and actually help the cord to rot off. If you deliver your baby at home, don't worry if the smell from the cord is offensive; the cord will fall off in 3 to 10 days. Keeping it outside the diaper is helpful. If signs of infection occur around the navel (heat, redness, tenderness, baby cries when touched) seek medical help.

BABY'S SKIN: Usually the newborn's skin peels off after a bit; that's natural. The skin can use some oiling with a natural oil (wheat germ oil, or half-and-half lanolin and safflower oil) but doesn't really need much washing except in the diaper area and around the neck. Careful attention to the diaper area will help prevent diaper rash. The few baths necessary in the first month might well be given to the baby while the mother is in the tub. Breast feeding at this time can help the baby to get used to the water. Pimples and "rashes" sometimes emerge on the skin as the sweat glands develop; unless they persist, don't worry about them.

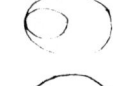

IRON: At around 3 months, a dip will occur in the baby's iron supplies. Commercial supplements of iron can permanently stain the baby teeth, so it's a good idea to start supplying the little one with supplementary liquids or foods. Since these take longer to digest than milk, they will also help establish sleep patterns. The following are good supplements, high in iron and minerals.

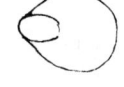

APRICOTS: dried apricots can be covered with water and soaked overnight; you can feed the juice to the baby and eat the apricots yourself. When the baby is ready for food, you can grind them in a blender or Happy Baby Food Grinder (wonderful to have. Order from Bowland Jacobs Co., Spring Valley, Ill.)

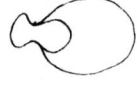

WAKAME SEAWEED: Take 3 inches of seaweed and pour 1 cup of boiling water over it -- soak for 20 minutes and feed water to baby. When baby begins to eat solids, you can mix the seaweed in with other vegetables like carrots, and blend or grind.

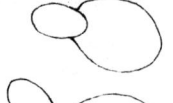

MISO SOUP: boil a cup of water. Mix a little boiling water with ½ tsp. miso and make a paste. Add remaining water, stir, and let sit a few minutes. Feed the broth to the baby.

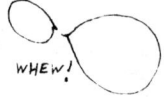
WHEW!

Other foods high in minerals are torula or brewer's yeast, blackstrap molasses, malt syrup, and Dr. Bronner's carrot syrup -- all of which are good to add to yogurt, but in small amounts as they are very laxative. (See also Page 57 on Iron, and Pages 16-17 on Babies and Small Children.

pregnancy & childbirth

nursing

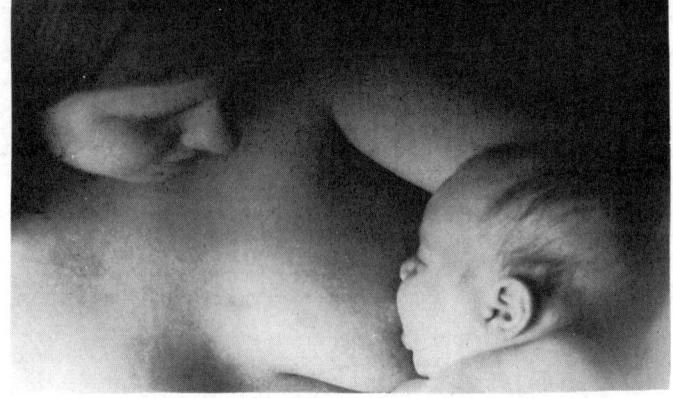

Don't forget that lactation demands <u>more</u> calories, minerals, and vitamins than pregnancy. (Please see pages 53-58 on Vitamins and Minerals.) You need 1000 more calories than normal, so this is not the time to try to lose weight by dieting. If you choose to nurse, try to tolerate some extra weight until the baby is weaned.

To strengthen your nipples, and avoid nursing problems, begin in your last month of pregnancy to massage the nipples with cocoa butter or wheat germ oil. Hold the alveola (the dark area of the breast) between the thumb and index finger, and rub the fingers back and forth, firmly. This should be done once or twice a day. When the baby's born, don't fall asleep nursing at first -- don't nurse too long on either side. Begin with 5 minutes on each side. Let your breasts gradually get accustomed to their new job. Then you can do whatever feels good.

For the first three days, your breasts will exude a yellow substance, colostrum, which provides your infant with the perfect food and antibodies to begin its new life. On the third day, your breasts will probably swell up like footballs, becoming very hard and probably quite painful. Your temperature may go up at this time. This is when the milk comes in. Many women have a desire to cry at this time, which is perfectly natural. It may be that the crying is a direct hormonal response to the milk coming in, and that the letting down of tears enables the milk to let down and flow into all the little milk ducts, like the spring rain flowing into all the dry gullies.

When you're engorged, you may want to use a breast pump or have someone suck your nipples to relieve the extreme pressure. This definitely eases the pain, and makes it easier for the baby to suck the breast, when it's not so engorged. Also, get plenty of fluids. Drink lots of milk (up to 6 cups a day). Engorgement is not affected by how much you drink. Drink freely, according to your thirst. For pain with engorgement, apply cold wash cloths, or an ice bag wrapped in a towel.

When nursing, watch your nipples closely, and at the first sign of DRYNESS or CRACKING, open Vitamin E capsules (a pin through both ends works well) and apply the oil to the nipples, several times a day. Wipe off the excess. Use a breast shield for awhile if necessary. At the first sign of RAW, TENDER nipples, mix 1/4 tsp. salt with 2 tsp.s warm water and apply to nipples. It will sting just a little, then you can literally feel the skin tightening up. Leave it on for 10 minutes, then wash it off (baby will scream if you don't).

TO DRY OUT YOUR MILK when you want to stop nursing, drink Sage Tea. Boil 1 cup of water and pour over 1 tsp. sage leaves -- brew 5 minutes. Drink freely.

Vitamins

The Minimum Daily requirements given here are for perfectly healthy people living in an environment without stress. Since this does not describe most people, it is up to you to adjust your intake of all of these vitamins and minerals to meet your own needs.

Vitamin A — fat soluble

Minimum Daily Requirements:
Lactating Women: 8,000 U.S.P. Units
Pregnant Women: 6,000 U.S.P. Units
Men, Women, Boys, Girls: 5,000 U.S.P. Units
Children: 2,500 U.S.P. Units

NOTE: During illness the need for Vitamin A is increased because absorption is poor and the storage of Vitamin A in the liver is impaired.

Foods Highest In Vitamin A (over 5,000 units)

fish liver oil, livers, beet green, broccoli, carrots, cauliflower, swiss chard, collard greens, dandelion greens, endive, kale, lamb's quarters, loose leaf lettuce, mustard greens, spinach, winter squash, sweet potatoes, tomatoes, turnip greens, watercress, apricots, cantaloupe, cherries, papayas, peaches, persimmons, prunes

What Vitamin A Does For You

Builds resistance to INFECTIONS, especially of the respiratory tract. Permits formation of visual purple in the eye, counteracting NIGHT BLINDNESS, weak EYESIGHT, and LIGHT SENSITIVITY. Promotes healthy SKIN. Essential for PREGNANCY and LACTATION. Increases LONGEVITY and delays SENILITY.

What A Lack Of Vitamin A Does To You

NIGHT BLINDNESS. LIGHT SENSITIVITY. Increased susceptibility to INFECTIONS. Dry, scaly, or oily SKIN. Defective TEETH having a thin and weak enamel. Retarded GROWTH.

NOTE: ANTACID PILLS, when taken in excess, neutralize the hydrochloric acid in the stomach, making it difficult to break down fats, including the fat-soluble vitamins. This would impair absorption of Vitamins A, D, and K. Instead of antacid pills, we recommend slippery elm, as described on page 8 for Gas. The powdered slippery elm may be taken in "00" caps and 2 caps may be swallowed down with hot water or tea, whenever needed. MINERAL OIL (vaseline, baby oil, and many cosmetic oils) is taken into the body, whether used internally or externally. Once inside the body it can trap your fat-soluble vitamins. Then, since the body doesn't absorb the mineral oil, the vitamins will be excreted along with the oil. Anyone showing deficiency symptoms of Vitamin A should use only natural oils on their skin. Vegetable oils or wheat germ oil may be substituted. FLUORESCENT LIGHTING, after prolonged exposure, can cause your Vitamin A needs to increase rapidly. CONTACT LENSES also may increase your body's use of and thus need for Vitamin A.

Other Nutrients Needed For Best Absorption Of Vitamin A

VITAMIN E is necessary for proper absorption of Vitamin A. FAT is also required, because the fat-soluble vitamins will not be absorbed without it, so when eating foods or supplements high in Vitamins A, D, or E, be sure to include at the same meal butter, margarine, mayonnaise, oil, whole milk, avocadoes, or other sources of fat. IF FAT-SOLUBLE VITAMINS ARE TAKEN BETWEEN MEALS, IT'S ADVISABLE TO WASH THEM DOWN WITH WHOLE MILK, INSTEAD OF WATER OR JUICE. If there's a disease of the GALL BLADDER, there won't be enough bile to break down the Vitamin A, so if there are signs of a Vitamin A deficiency, bile tablets and lecithin should be used.

Effects Of Excessive Intake Of Vitamin A

Thinning HAIR. Sore LIPS. BRUISING. NOSEBLEEDS. HEADACHES. Blurred VISION. Flaking itching SKIN. Painful JOINTS and tenderness and swelling over the long BONES. (Seen in people taking 100,000 to 500,000 units a day for over a year.) Lab experiments with animals have shown Vitamin A overdose during a critical period in pregnancy to be one of the factors that can result in a cleft palate in offspring. Oddly enough, the same symptoms will sometimes result when the mother animal's diet is deficient in Vitamin A.

NOTE: Toxicity can be prevented by getting adequate Vitamin C.

B Vitamins
water soluble

The B Vitamins work together, as a team. If you get an excess of one B vitamin, it can cause the body to excrete the B Vitamins that are then relatively deficient. (Apparently Vitamin B_3, Niacin, is the one B Vitamin that can be taken alone without throwing the others others off balance.) This is the danger of taking any of the individual B Vitamins. Unfortunately, it is a problem even with the better B Complex supplements, because folic acid and PABA (members of the B family) are regulated by the Food and Drug Administration, and the amounts allowed are so small that it completely unbalances the proportions of the other B Vitamins. Folic acid is regulated because it masks pernicious anemia (Vitamin B_{12} deficiency), and thus vegetarians could come down with pernicious anemia without even knowing it. Of course, this could easily be remedied simply by including Vitamin B_{12} in any supplement that contains folic acid -- but they apparently haven't thought of that. PABA is regulated because it is a sulfa drug suppressant. This regulation dates back to the days when sulfa drugs were far more widespread than they are today.

This is why we feel that the best way to get B Vitamins is by making them a part of your diet by eating at least 1 Tbsp. of yogurt every day, drinking milk, and eating vegetables with roughage to keep your yogurt colony going. And be sure to eat whole grains and avoid refined foods. If you really have signs of a B Vitamin deficiency, eat torula or brewer's yeast every day (at least 1 Tbsp.), and liver once a week, and wheat germ regularly.

If a supplement has to be taken, we recommend taking the whole B Complex in a supplement that has equal amounts of B_2 and B_6, even if you only seem to be short in one of the B's. But supplements should be taken only as a temporary remedy for stress, and *only* with ample amounts of yogurt, liver, wheat germ, brewer's yeast, and milk in the diet. One of the more balanced supplements is Plus Products Formula 71. If you want a supplement with more Niacin, try Formula 72.

B Vitamins should be taken before a meal, because they need to combine with food for maximum effectiveness. Or they can be taken with a snack, or just after a meal.

Coffee, alcohol, and diuretics wash out your B Vitamins.

Vitamin B_1 — Thiamine

Minimum Daily Requirements: Men, Nursing Mothers, Boys: 1.2 mg.s   Women: .8 mg.s
Girls, Pregnant Women: 1.0 mg.s   Children: .6 mg.s

Foods Highest In Vitamin B_1 (over 5 mgs.)
brewer's or torula yeast (1 tsp.), pork, organ meats, soy flour, brown rice, whole wheat flour (1 cup), wheat germ (1/3 cup), brazil nuts (1/2 cup), natural peanut butter (1/3 cup), sunflower seeds (3 Tbsps.)

What Vitamin B_1 Does For You
Promotes GROWTH, essential for normal functioning of NERVE TISSUES, MUSCLES, and HEART. Essential for DIGESTION.

What A Lack Of Vitamin B_1 Does To You
May lead to loss of APPETITE, WEAKNESS and lassitude, NERVOUS IRRITABILITY, INSOMNIA, loss of WEIGHT, vague ACHES AND PAINS, MENTAL DEPRESSION and CONSTIPATION. In children, it may impair GROWTH. In severe cases: BERIBERI. Since B_1 is essential for a healthy NERVOUS SYSTEM, a lack of it will manifest itself in a loss of ankle and knee jerk reflexes, neuritis, muscular weakness in the feet, calves and thighs. MENTAL SYMPTOMS would include mental instability, poor memory, vague fears, uneasiness, and ideas of persecution.

Vitamin B_2 — Riboflavin

Minimum Daily Requirements: Boys, Nursing Mothers: 1.8 mg.s   Women: 1.3 mg.s
Men: 1.7 mg.s   Children: 1.0 mg.s
Girls, Pregnant Women: 1.5 mg.s

Foods Highest In Vitamin B_2 (over 5 mgs.)
livers, kidney, milk (1 cup), brewer's yeast (2 Tbsp.s), torula yeast (1 tsp.), cottage cheese, turnip greens, macaroni and cheese, wheat germ (1 cup), almonds (1/2 cup)

What Vitamin B_2 Does For You
Improves GROWTH, essential for healthy EYES, SKIN, AND MOUTH. Promotes general HEALTH. Important for RESPIRATION.

What A Lack Of Vitamin B_2 Does To You
May result in itching and burning of EYES, bloodshot eyes, cataracts, dimness of vision. Cracking of corners of LIPS, inflammation or sores on the MOUTH, purplish tongue, inflammation at tip and margin of tongue. Degeneration of NERVOUS TISSUES, resulting in loss of coordination, MENTAL CONFUSION, and loss of MUSCULAR STRENGTH in the ARMS and LEGS.

Vitamin B$_3$ — Niacin

Niacinamide is more generally used since it minimizes the burning, flushing, and itching of the skin that frequently occurs with Niacin (Nicotinic Acid).

Minimum Daily Requirements:
- Pregnant Women: 21 mg.s
- Boys, Nursing Mothers: 20 mg.s
- Men: 19 mg.s
- Girls: 17 mg.s
- Women: 14 mg.s
- Children: 11 mg.s

Foods Highest In Vitamin B$_3$ (over 2.5 mgs.)
meat, poultry, organ meats, fish (with the <u>exception</u> of clams, fish sticks, lobster, oyster stew, scallops, shrimp), mushrooms, dried apricots, dried dates, bran flakes, brown or converted rice, rice polish, wheat germ (1 cup), whole wheat (cooked, 1/2 cup), peanut butter (natural unhydrogenated, 2 Tbsp.s), peanuts (2 Tbsp.s), sunflower seeds (2 Tbsp.s), brewer's yeast (1 Tbsp.), torula yeast (1 tsp.)

What Vitamin B$_3$ Does For You
Especially important for the proper functioning of the NERVOUS SYSTEM. Promotes GROWTH. Maintains normal function of the GASTRO-INTESTINAL tract. Necessary for metabolism of SUGAR. Helps maintain normal SKIN condition.

What A Lack Of Vitamin B$_3$ Does To You
Sore TONGUE. Dysfunction of the NERVOUS SYTEM. MENTAL DEPRESSION and IRRITABILITY. Fatigue HEADACHES and vague ACHES and PAINS. Loss of APPETITE and WEIGHT. NAUSEA, VOMITING, and ABDOMINAL PAINS. Mental symptoms ranging from loss of MEMORY to STUPOR or MANIA. PELLAGRA: a disease characterized by the above symptoms and caused by vitamin deficiency, mostly of niacin and Vitamin B2. Begins with an inflamed mouth and the tongue red and sore -- then cracks and sores appear in the skin around the mouth.

NOTE: A dietary deficiency of niacin is usually accompanied by deficiencies of B$_1$, B$_2$ and B$_6$.

Vitamin B$_6$ — Pyridoxine

Minimum Daily Requirements: 5-10 mg.s

Foods Highest In Vitamin B$_6$
meat, fish, wheat germ, egg yolk, cantaloupe, cabbage, milk, yeast, whole grains, organ meats

What Vitamin B$_6$ Does For You
Aids in FOOD ASSIMILATION and in protein and fat metabolism. Prevents various NERVOUS disorders, SKIN disorders, and NAUSEA.

What A Lack Of Vitamin B$_6$ Does To You
May result in NERVOUSNESS, INSOMNIA, SKIN eruptions, including ECZEMA, loss of MUSCLE CONTROL, VOMITING, GAS, DIARRHEA, CANCERS.

NOTE: PREGNANT WOMEN are notoriously deficient in B$_6$. STREPTOMYCIN appears to destroy B$_6$, or to increase the need for it, thus sometimes causing epileptic-like convulsions in children.

Other Nutrients Needed For Best Absorption: magnesium

Vitamin B$_{12}$ — Cobalamin

Minimum Daily Requirements: 1-3 micrograms (mcg.s)

Foods Highest In Vitamin B$_{12}$
liver, beef, pork, eggs, milk, cheese, fish, organ meats, yeast, wheat germ, soy beans

NOTE: this is the vitamin that strict VEGETARIANS are in danger of being in need of. But it's hard to detect a B$_{12}$ deficiency in a vegetarian because of the high folic acid content of the blood. Nerve damage can therefore occur before the deficiency is detected, so strict vegetarians have been advised to take 1 tablet (50 micrograms) of B$_{12}$ each week.

What Vitamin B$_{12}$ Does For You
Helps in the formation and regeneration of RED BLOOD CELLS, thus helping to prevent ANEMIA. Promotes GROWTH and increased APPETITE in children. A general TONIC for adults.

What A Lack Of Vitamin B$_{12}$ Does To You
May lead to nutritional and pernicious ANEMIAS, TIREDNESS, poor APPETITE and GROWTH failure in children. Vegetarians often develop these symptoms: sore MOUTHS and TONGUES, MENSTRUAL disturbances, NERVE disorders: "needles and pins" feeling in hands and feet, neuritis, pain and stiffness in spine, difficulty in walking.

Other Nutrients Needed For Best Absorption Of Vitamin B$_{12}$
Vitamin B$_6$, Vitamin C, adequate protein

Vitamin C

water soluble

MINIMUM DAILY REQUIREMENTS: when NOT under stress: Boys, Girls: 80 mg.s
Pregnant women, Nursing mothers: 100 mg.s   Men, Women: 70 mg.s

Foods Highest In Vitamin C (over 25 mgs.)

the following steamed vegetables: beet greens, broccoli, brussel sprouts, cabbage (or raw), cauliflower, collards, dandelion greens, kale, lamb's quarters, mustard greens, spinach, turnip greens, turnips-- also raw kohlrabi, raw green peppers, tomatoes, livers, raw watercress, cantaloupe, papaya, rose hips, acerola cherries, citrus fruits

What Vitamin C Does For You

Necessary for healthy TEETH, GUMS, and BONES, strengthens all connective tissue, promotes WOUND healing, maintains CAPILLARY walls, helps maintain sound HEALTH and ENERGY. DETOXIFIES the body, thus giving protection when potentially harmful drugs or X-rays must be taken.

What A Lack Of Vitamin C Does To You

May lead to soft and bleeding GUMS, TOOTH decay, loss of APPETITE, MUSCULAR weakness, BRUISES, capillary weakness, ANEMIA, NOSEBLEEDS, HEMORRHAGES.
NOTE: during an INFECTION, Vitamin C is quickly destroyed in the body, and so the body's need for Vitamin C rises dramatically according to the seriousness of the infection. Also, Vitamin C reacts with any foreign substance reaching the blood, so that more Vitamin C is destroyed by drugs and hence more is required while taking drugs. Also, during STRESS, harmful substances are formed in the body -- once again, Vitamin C can detoxify these substances if enough is supplied, but then it is used up and carried away in the urine and so the need for Vitamin C is increased. Also, each CIGARETTE destroys about 25 mg.s of Vitamin C.

Other Nutrients Needed For Best Absorption Of Vitamin C

pantothenic acid (member of the B complex), Vitamin B6

Effects Of Excessive Intake Of Vitamin C

DIARRHEA, RASH - caused by the acetone (airplane glue) in ascorbic acid pills.

Vitamin D

fat soluble

MINIMUM DAILY REQUIREMENTS: everyone: 400 USP units
NOTE: The need for Vitamin D increases for adolescent girls, people with porous bones (old people), and during illness or stress.

Foods Highest In Vitamin D

sunlight, fish-liver oils, eggs, Vitamin D fortified milk products, bone meal, organ meats, fish (especially cod, herring, tuna, sardines, and salmon).
NOTE: Vitamin D is formed in the oil on the skin by summer sunshine. Winter sun produces no Vitamin D. And the oil on the skin washes off with water, even cold water.

What Vitamin D Does For You

Regulates the use of CALCIUM and PHOSPHORUS in the body and is therefore necessary for the proper formation of BONES and TEETH. Essential for preventing RICKETS (softening of the BONES in children, with the result of bow-legs or other mis-shaped bones). Important for GROWTH, VIGOR and development during infancy and childhood.

What A Lack Of Vitamin D Does To You

May lead to various SKELETAL deformities, such as bow-legs, knock-knees, enlargement of the ends of the long bones, curvature of the spine, softening of the skull and delayed closing of the anterior fontanelle in infants. TOOTH DECAY. Retarded GROWTH and lack of VIGOR. MUSCULAR weakness. Enlarged PARATHYROID glands. Low serum calcium and low body phosphorus.
NOTE: Rickets is now uncommon in the United States because of Vitamin D enriched milk. But dark-skinned people would tend to be more vulnerable to it, since the pigment in dark skin blocks absorption of the sun's rays. Especially living in a place like Seattle, where there's not much sun during most of the year. If a dark-skinned person is also allergic to milk (see Page on Diarrhea), the problem becomes much more serious and we would recommend using Vitamin A and calcium supplements. Please see also page 53 on fat-soluble vitamins.

Effects Of Excessive Intake Of Vitamin D

WEAKNESS, VOMITING, DIARRHEA, HEADACHES, demineralization of BONES, and calcification of soft tissues; MUSCLE SPASM, inflammation of the PANCREAS, CONVULSIONS, a kind of DIABETES, HYPERTENSION, irreversible KIDNEY damage, even DEATH (with 100,000 to 500,000 units daily). With INFANTS, 1800 units can inhibit growth. If taken during PREGNANCY, infants may have badly shaped jaws with a faulty bite, be mentally defective, or suffer obstruction of blood flow.
NOTE: Vitamin D toxicity can be prevented with adequate Vitamin C, A and choline.

Vitamin E (fat soluble)

Vitamin E requirement is unusually high in men during the reproductive age, women after menopause, and all obese people. Vitamin E is sold as mixed tocopherols or as d-alpha tocopherols. Research indicates that only the alpha tocopherol can function as a vitamin, so that is the kind we recommend. Vitamin E is never toxic. The MDR for Vitamin E has not been established.

Foods Highest In Vitamin E
uncooked wheat germ oil, whole-grain breads and cereals, margarine, eggs, organ meats
NOTE: it's difficult to get enough Vitamin E in your diet, so we do recommend taking supplements. Also, BREAST MILK from healthy mothers usually contains 20 times as much Vitamin E as cow's milk.

What Vitamin E Does For You
ANTIOXIDANT: when the following nutrients in the body are exposed to oxygen coming into the body, unless there is adequate Vitamin E in the body, they will be destroyed: essential fatty acids, carotene, Vitamin A, B Vitamins (indirectly), and the pituitary, adrenal, and sex hormones. Vitamin E is necessary for normal REPRODUCTION and in helping to prevent sterility (see above). Helps prevent MISCARRIAGES. Prevents CALCIUM DEPOSITS in blood vessel walls. Valuable in treatment of HEART conditions and cardio-vascular diseases. Strengthens capillary walls and thus decreases CLOTTING. Reduces the body's need for OXYGEN. Acts as a regulator of the METABOLISM of the cell nucleus. Helps prevent or remove SCARRING.

What A Lack Of Vitamin E Does To You
Loss of REPRODUCTIVE powers. MUSCULAR disorders. IRON absorption and hemoglobin formation are impaired. RED BLOOD CELLS become fragile. Since Vitamin E protects the essential fatty acids from destruction by oxygen, a lack of Vitamin E will result in the essential fatty acids being destroyed. And since they are a part of the cell structure, a lack of Vitamin E can result in clot formation. NERVOUSNESS. General WEAKNESS.
NOTE: 90% of Vitamin E in oils is destroyed by cooking. Vitamin E is also destroyed by taking iron salts, by exposure to air, by radiation, and by X-rays. Also, the more oil or fat you eat the more Vitamin E you need.

Other Nutrients Needed For Best Absorption Of Vitamin E
Vitamin C
Also, please see page 53 on Vitamin A, under the same category, for notes on oil soluble vitamins.

Minerals

Iron

Minimum Daily Requirements:
Pregnant Women, Nursing Mothers: 20 mg.s   Men, Children: 10 mg.s
Women, Boys, Girls: 15 mg.s

Foods Highest In Iron (over 5 mgs.)
organ meats, clams, oysters, dulse seaweed (2/3 tsp.), kelp (1 tsp.), irish moss or agar seaweed (4 tbsp.s), red kidney beans, soybeans, steamed dandelion greens, dried or canned apricots, prune juice, rice polish (1/3 cup), wheat germ (1 cup), sesame seeds (1/2 cup -- try them pan roasted or ground; raw whole seeds won't digest unless you're a religious chewer), brewer's yeast (3 tbsp.s), blood (Blood is THE BEST source of iron, and our prudish dietary customs should not rule it out. Blood sausage, black puddings, etc. are available (but be sure not to get ordinary supermarket ones full of preservatives). If you can get straight blood, it's great fried.).
NOTE: Iron supplements are not recommended, but if taken they should be followed 12 hours later by 100 International units of Vitamin E.

What Iron Does For You
Iron is needed by the body to make hemoglobin, which is the component in red blood cells which carries OXYGEN to each cell; oxygen is required for all bodily processes, particularly ENERGY.

What A Lack Of Iron Does To You
A constant feeling of TIREDNESS: lack of endurance. A pale COMPLEXION. Shortness of BREATH. Possibly DIZZINESS. HEADACHES. MENTAL DEPRESSION.

Other Nutrients Needed For Best Absorption Of Iron
Vitamin B6, Vitamin C, magnesium

CALCIUM

Minimum Daily Requirements: Boys: 1400 mg.s   Children, Men: 800 mg.s
Girls, Pregnant Women, Nursing Mothers: 1300 mg.s

Foods Highest In Calcium (over 300 mgs.)

milk (1 cup), cheddar cheese, swiss cheese, sardines, kelp (1 oz. or 2 tbsp.s), Irish moss seaweed or agar (3 tbsp.s), the following steamed vegetables: collard greens, dandelion greens, lambs quarters, mustard greens, trunip greens -- macaroni and cheese, dry sesame seeds (1/3 cup -- try them panroasted or ground; raw whole seeds won't digest unless you're a religious chewer), molasses (3 tbsp.s), calcium - fortified torula yeast (2 tbsp.s), bone meal or powder, calcium glucouate, calcium lactate, dicalcium phosphate. If a supplement is needed, you can try A.D.L. CAL-MAG liquid. It contains calcium. magnesium and Vitamin D.

What Calcium Does For You

Builds and maintains BONES and TEETH. Helps BLOOD to clot. Aids VITALITY and endurance. Regulates HEART rhythm. Maintains MUSCLE tone.

What A Lack Of Calcium Does To You

TENSION, NERVOUSNESS, HEADACHES, INSOMNIA, MENTAL DEPRESSION, WATER RETENTION, low RESISTANCE, MUSCLE cramps. (All of the above have been associated with Menstrual "blues" -- please see also page 38 on Women: Cramps.)

NOTES: PREGNANT WOMEN and CHILDREN, particularly should probably avoid the following COOKED GREENS: spinach, beet greens, dock, and sorrel -- the oxalic acid released in the cooking interferes with calcium and possibly iron absorption. Calcium absorption is also said to be impaired by eating CHOCOLATE.

Other Nutrients Needed For Best Absorption Of Calcium

magnesium (You need about half as much magnesium as calcium - if you get more than half as much magnesium, it will create a calcium deficiency.), protein, B Vitamins, Vitamin C, Vitamin D, estrogen

Effects Of Excessive Intake Of Calcium

When calcium is taken in large amounts without the above nutrients, too much magnesium is excreted, resulting in DIARRHEA, (as with some bottle-fed babies or ulcer patients), or KIDNEY STONES. Phosphorus is also lost. Calcium may be deposited in joints and/or veins.

MAGNESIUM

average intake appears to be only half the adult requirement. Food grown in soil treated with lime or with chemical fertilizers containing potassium do not have much magnesium or trace elements. If you have a garden, we recommend using Dolomite instead of lime, and compost or organic fertilizers instead of chemical fertilizers.

Minimum Daily Requirements: Pregnant Women, Nursing Mothers: 450 mg.s   Children: 200 mg.s
Men, Women, Boys, Girls: 350 mg.s

Foods Highest In Magnesium (over 100 mgs.)

soy flour (1/3 cup), whole wheat flour (1 cup), raisin bran (1 cup), wheat bran (1½ tbsp.s), wheat germ (5 tbsp.s), blackstrap molasses (2 tbsp.s), kelp (1 tbsp.s), dried or toasted almonds (¼ cup), brazil nuts (2½ tbsp.s), cashews (½ cup), peanuts (¼ cup), dry sesame seeds (¼ cup - see note under calcium), steamed swiss chard (1 cup), steamed collard greens (1 cup) -- may also be taken as a supplement in the form of magnesium oxide, which contains 250 mg.s per tablet or ¼ tsp. A good supplement is A.D.L. CAL-MAG, which contains calcium, magnesium and Vitamin D.

What Magnesium Does For You

Maintains normal function of the BRAIN, SPINAL CORD, and all NERVES.

Magnesium Does To You

DIARRHEA. TREMORS. MUSCLE SPASMS of the arms, hands, legs, feet and eyes, or epileptic-like convulsions. PSYCHOSIS.

NOTE: Magnesium is lost rapidly when drinking ALCOHOL, or eating REFINED FOODS, SUBARS, and HYDROGENATED FATS.

Other Nutrients Needed For Best Absorption Of Magnesium

protein, calcium (magnesium intake should be about half that of calcium -- if calcium intake is _more_ than twice as high as magnesium, a magnesium deficiency will occur

Effects Of Excessive Intake Of Magnesium

Excessive magnesium will hoard the available albumin, crowding out the CALCIUM and causing it to be lost in the urine.

Home Remedy Self-Help Kit

When you're sick, you don't really want to start running around to health food stores and herb stores, looking for "home remedies". And you surely don't want to begin then to prepare medications that take a week to make! And so, in order for the remedies mentioned in this little book to become truly home remedies for you, we've compiled a list of herbs and other medications which together would make up a very useful First Aid Kit. After each item, we give a list of the ailments that we've recommended this item to be used for // and something about how each one works. You can choose the ones you feel would be most appropriate for your family's needs. The quantities given are suggested minimums for a family of 4-6. (Underlined words are explained at the end of the First Aid Pages, page 63.)

HERBS

ALOE VERA GEL -- 2 oz. bottle of gel OR a medium to large-sized plant (the gel from the leaves may be used fresh, or boil to the consistency of thick honey and let cool and pour into a jar; it will solidify) -- used for burns (also heals cuts and wounds)

BEARBERRY LEAF (UVA URSI) -- ½ oz. -- used for bladder infections (also good in smoking mixture) // astringent, diuretic, tonic

BURDOCK ROOT -- ½ oz. -- used for all kinds of skin problems // tones up organs secreting impurities from the blood (kidneys, lungs, liver, lymph glands), diuretic

CATNIP LEAF -- 1 oz. -- used for headaches, insomnia, nervousness (also good for colic) // reduces nerve sensitivity, nervine, relieves spasms, induces perspiration and stimulates blood flow, stimulates gastro-intestinal mucous membrane, carminative

CAYENNE POWDER (CAPSICUM) -- 1 oz. -- used for coughs, in lower bowel tonic, for diarrhea, in liniment for aches and pains, stomach flu, difficulty eating, upset stomach after meals // astringent, stimulates gastro-intestinal mucous membrane, promotes secretion of saliva, prevents or relieves vomiting, stops decay of cells and formation of pus (high in sulfur), reduces or relieves spasms, carminative, stimulates profuse sweating when taken hot, good for the heart, excites and increases nervous sensibility, does not accelerate the pulse, equalizes and restores balance of circulation in all parts, increases secretions in the stomach and strengthens and tonifies its movements, tonic // NOT RECOMMENDED FOR PEOPLE WITH STOMACH ULCERS

CINNAMON (CASSIA BARK) -- 1 oz. -- we recommend Saigon or Ceylon Cinnamon, but any kind will do -- used for diarrhea, stomach pain, stomach flu // stimulates increased secretions in stomach; tonifies and strengthens its movements. carminative, mild astringent

COLTSFOOT LEAVES -- 1 oz. - used for coughs, asthma, headaches // demulcent, expectorant, tonic

COMFREY ROOT -- 1 oz. -- used for asthma, coughs, diarrhea, menstrual cramps, sore throats (also used as poultice to help mend broken bones and reduce swelling) // mild astringent, demulcent, clears out phlegm from chest or lungs, expectorant, high in calcium and allantoin (strengthens epithelial formations) // DON'T MIX WITH CHAMOMILE because it destroys the allantoin

CORNSILK (from Indian corn) -- ½ oz. -- used for asthma and for bladder infections // reduces nerve sensitivity, diuretic, stimulates kidneys, tones up organs secreting impurities from blood (kidneys, lungs, liver, lymph glands)

ECHINACEA ROOT -- 1 oz. -- used for strep, staph, bladder infections // tones up organs secreting impurities from blood (kidneys, lungs, liver, lymph glands), stimulates and cleanses lymph glands, stops decay of cells and formation of pus (high in sulfur), facili-

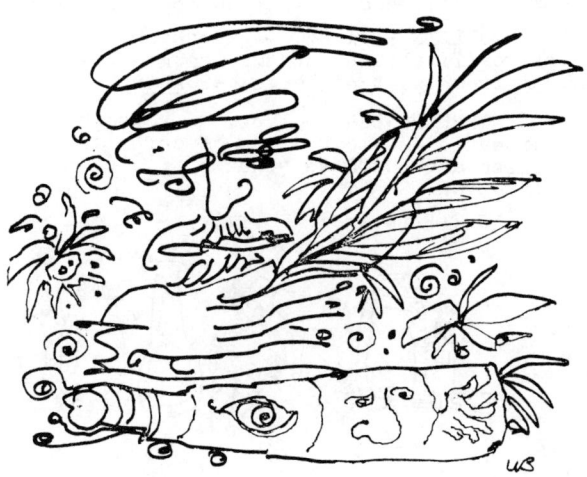

[59]

HOME REMEDY SELF-HELP KIT

page two

tates the elimination of toxins from the organism, and has a destructive effect upon streptococci and staphylococci.

ELDER FLOWERS -- 1/2 oz. -- used for fever, diarrhea // <u>alterative</u>, increases the secretion and regulates the flow of urine, <u>expectorant</u>, mild laxative, opens the pores and stimulates free perspiration, <u>diuretic</u>

EPHEDRA -- 1 oz. -- used for asthma, sinus congestion, nasal congestion, chest congestion // <u>nervine</u>, reduces or relieves spasms, <u>expectorant</u>, clears out phlegm from chest or lungs, acts on air passages

GENTIAN ROOT -- 1/2 oz. -- for nausea, lack of appetite, upset stomach after meals // relieves biliousness, <u>tonic</u>, stimulates gastrointestinal mucous membrane, stimulates increased secretions in stomach and strengthens and tonifies its movements, stops decay of cells and formation of pus, high in sulfur

GOLDEN SEAL ROOT, POWDER -- 2 oz. -- used for sore throats, in lower bowel tonic, in liniment for aches and pains, hepatitis, stomach pain, stomach flu, lack of appetite, upset stomach after meals, mouth rinse for gum diseases, bladder infections // stimulates and cleanses lymphatic glands, tones up organs secreting impurities from blood (kidneys, liver, lungs, lymph glands), stops decay of cells and formation of pus, high in sulfur, <u>laxative</u>, relaxes and removes obstructions from alimentary canal, <u>diuretic</u>, <u>tonic</u>, stimulates secretions of stomach and tonifies and strengthens its movements, <u>astringent</u>, soothing to mucous membranes, stimulates the gastrointestinal mucous membranes

HOREHOUND -- 1/4 oz. -- used for persistent coughs // stimulates gastrointestinal mucous membranes, induces perspiration, opens pores, stimulates blood flow, causes increased flow of bile from liver, <u>expectorant</u>, clears out phlegm from chest or lungs, <u>tonic</u>, <u>diuretic</u>

JUNIPER BERRIES -- 1/4 oz. -- used for bladder infections // <u>diuretic</u>, influences kidneys, stimulates increased secretions in stomach and strengthens and tonifies its movements, <u>carminative</u>

LOBELIA LEAF -- 1/2 oz. -- used for asthma // <u>expectorant</u>, induces vomiting (taken in excess), relieves spasms, <u>nervine</u>, induces perspiration and stimulates blood flow, <u>diuretic</u>

MOTHERWORT -- 1/2 oz. -- used for cramps (IUD or menstrual) // reduces or relieves spasms, influences liver and causes increased flow of bile, <u>nervine</u>, laxative, promotes menstruation, good to take during pregnancy

MULLEIN -- 1 oz. -- used for asthma, coughs, sore throat, runny nose, diarrhea // <u>astringent</u>, relieves spasms, counteracts dryness, reduces itching and pain, clears out phlegm from chest or lungs, <u>diuretic</u>

MYRRH POWDER -- 1 oz. -- sore throats, liniment for aches and pains, mouth rinse for gum diseases // stops decay of cells and formation of pus (high in sulfur), <u>expectorant</u>, equalizes and restores balance of circulation in all parts of the body, <u>tonic</u>, promotes menstruation

NETTLE (stinging nettle) -- 1 oz. -- used for asthma, diarrhea, pubic hair itching,

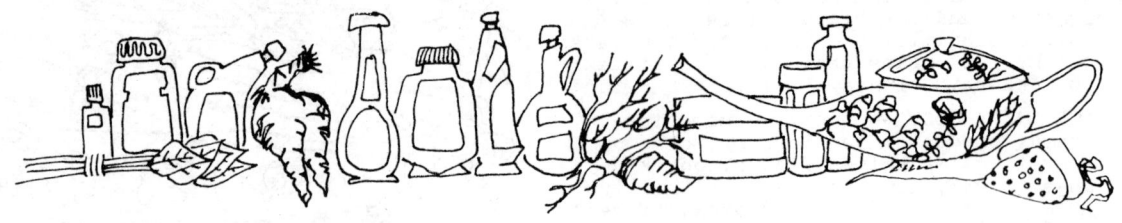

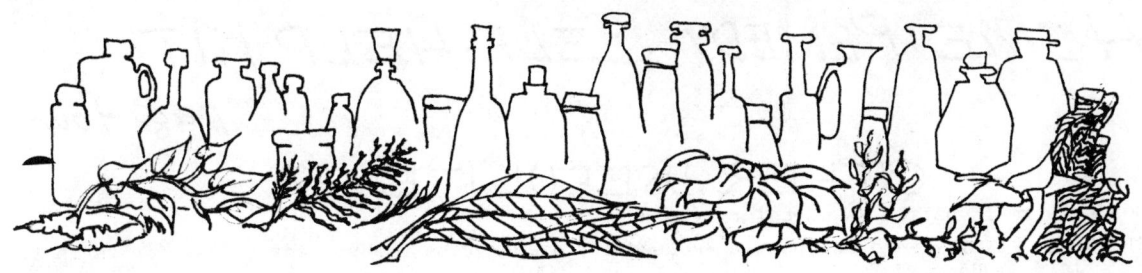

Home Remedy Self-Help Kit
page three

Nettle (cont.) dandruff and other hair problems // <u>astringent</u>, influences kidneys, clears out phlegm from chest or lungs, <u>tonic</u>, <u>diuretic</u>

PARSLEY -- 1/2 oz. -- used for toxemia // <u>diuretic</u>, mild laxative, <u>carminative</u>, <u>expectorant</u>, <u>tonic</u>, good for spleen and gall bladder

PEPPERMINT -- 2 oz. -- used to flavor other teas, good for stomach, for fevers, diarrhea, headaches, nausea, to stop vomiting // reduces fever by stimulating profuse sweating and enhancing evaporation, prevents griping, reduces or relieves spasms, <u>carminative</u>, <u>nervine</u>, reduces nervous energy, gives energy by equalizing and restoring the balance of circulation in all parts, increases secretions in stomach and strengthens and tonifies its movements, promotes menstruation

RASPBERRY LEAF TEA (Red Raspberry) -- 1/2 oz. -- used for cramps (IUD and menstrual) and as a tonic during pregnancy // gives strength and said to render childbirth easy and speedy, tones up organs secreting impurities from the blood (kidneys, lungs, liver, lymph glands), <u>astringent</u>, prevents or relieves vomiting, laxative, gives energy, equalizes and restores balance of circulation in all parts, stimulates secretions in stomach and strengthens and tonifies its movements, <u>tonic</u>

SAGE -- 1/2 oz. -- used for coughs, headaches, colds, dries out milk in nursing women, fevers // <u>astringent</u>, stimulates gastrointestinal mucous membrane, expels worms from stomach and intestines, reduces or relieves spasms, <u>nervine</u>, <u>expectorant</u>, stimulates sweat glands, <u>tonic</u>

SLIPPERY ELM -- (powdered or granulated) 1 oz. -- used for colic, mild laxative, sore throat, genital itching, nourishment during nausea or vomiting, nasal congestion, pubic hair itching, gas, stomach pain, stomach flu, stomach ulcers // <u>demulcent</u>, soothes skin, counteracts dryness, reduces itching and pain, soothes inflamed parts, nutritive, <u>diuretic</u>, clears out phlegm from chest or lungs, <u>astringent</u>

VALERIAN ROOT (in pieces or powdered) -- 1/2 oz. -- used for headaches, tension, insomnia // reduces nerve sensitivity, stimulates gastrointestinal mucous membrane, reduces or relieves spasms, <u>nervine</u>, equalizes and restores balance of circulation in all parts, <u>tonic</u>

YARROW FLOWERS -- 1/2 oz. -- used for bladder infections, cough syrup // stimulates and cleanses lymph glands, tones up organs secreting impurities from blood: kidneys, liver, lungs, lymph glands; <u>diuretic</u>, <u>tonic</u>, induces perspiration and stimulates blood flow

HOME REMEDY SELF-HELP KIT
page four

OTHER USEFUL ITEMS

ALCOHOL -- small bottle -- used for fevers

APPLE CIDER VINEGAR -- 8 oz. bottle -- used for diaper rash, to prevent colds, for vaginal infections

CALMS -- bottle of 100 -- used for nervousness, tension, and insomnia for adults and children. ($2.25 from Los Angeles Homeopathic Co., P. O. Box 61067, Los Angeles, California 90061 plus 35¢ handling)

CASTOR OIL -- 1 oz. bottle -- used for bruises, "black eyes"

CORN STARCH -- 1 box -- used for diaper rash, infection of foreskin, genital itching, heat rash

EUCALYPTUS OIL -- 1 oz. bottle -- used in steam for nasal congestion, asthma

GARLIC, ORGANIC -- plenty of it -- used to prevent colds, for toothaches, pinworms, coughs, sore throats, vaginal infections

HONEY -- at least two pounds -- used for coughs, burns, as a sweetener and preserver

HYDROGEN PEROXIDE -- small bottle -- to clean wounds, as a mouth rinse for gum disease

LEMON -- whole, or bottled juice -- used for coughs and sore throats and to help prevent colds

LINIMENT -- small bottle -- used for aches and pains, bangs and bumps (prepare yourself, according to instructions of page on Aches and Pains--do it now because it takes seven days)

OIL OF BITTER ORANGE -- 1/4 oz. bottle -- used for strep and staph (50¢ from Nature's Herb Co., 281 Ellis Street, San Francisco, California 94102, plus 25¢ postage)

00 GELATIN CAPSULES -- box of 100 -- for ease in swallowing hot or bitter herbs in powdered form

PEPPERMINT OIL -- 1 oz. bottle -- used for headaches

PYRINATE A200 -- small bottle -- used for crabs, lice, and scabies (or Kwell shampoo, if you have a prescription)

THOUSAND YEAR OLD EGGS -- 3-12 -- used for strep and middle ear infections (see pages on sore throats)

TIGER BALM -- one small vial -- used for sinus congestion, nasal congestion, chest congestion aches and pains (where Chinese items are sold)

TYLENOL -- small bottle -- used for teething and toothaches

VEGETABLE OIL (soy or safflower or all blend) -- 8 oz. bottle -- used for cradle cap, to prevent burning with garlic poultice or garlic suppositories, for nutrition in the Sorcerer's Potion given for hepatitis, for cooking as a healthful substitute for animal fats

WHEAT GERM OIL -- 2 oz. bottle -- (or open vitamin E oil capsules with a pin) -- used for diaper rash, herpes, pubic hair itching, burns, good for nipples of pregnant and nursing women, to prevent scarring and to speed healing

WITCH HAZEL -- small bottle -- used for herpes, mosquito bites, hemorrhoids

VITAMINS

VITAMINS A, B COMPLEX, C, D, AND E (Please see pages on vitamins for complete descriptions of these vitamins, their uses and natural food sources)

BREWER'S or TORULA YEAST -- 2 oz. -- used as an excellent source of B vitamins -- especially for hemorrhoids and also during pregnancy)

HOME REMEDY Self-help Kit

TERMINOLOGY

Usually we like to translate terminology into words that are understood by everybody. But in some cases, where one word wonderfully expresses a whole concept, we choose to retain the words and then try to define them. And so, for the words we've chosen to keep:

ASTRINGENTS: they stop excessive discharge by causing shrinkage of tissue. Useful for diarrhea, to reduce inflammation of mucous membranes (example: salt water gargle for sore throat), to stop bleeding, and to stop sweating. They will also restrain peristalsis (use <u>with</u> a carminative if you want to retain peristalsis)

CARMINATIVE: contains volatile oil - excites intestinal peristalsis - dispels gas from stomach and gastrointestinal tract - stimulates circulation - relaxes cardiac and pyloric orifices

DEMULCENT: soothes irritated mucous membranes to allow for healing (for example: comfrey root for stomach ulcers) and absorbs the discharge of pus through the skin

DIURETIC: increases the secretion and **stimulates the flow of urine** - stimulates the kidneys through the circulation **or the nervous system**

EXPECTORANT: encourages increased secretions and discharge from trachea, lungs and bronchi through coughing up

LAXATIVE: loosens without griping (cramping)

NERVINE: nerve tonic that rehabilitates and feeds the nerves. Mildly stimulating, yet lessens the excitement, irritability, or pain of the nervous system. Not to be confused with inorganic narcotics or opiates which attack and weaken the nerves

TONIC: herbs which give vitality and strength to the digestive system and related organs by stimulating nutrition. Sharpens the appetite and promotes better waste elimination, aids in digestion, and soothes the stomach. Usually bitter. Used in convalescence from diseases or any run-down condition

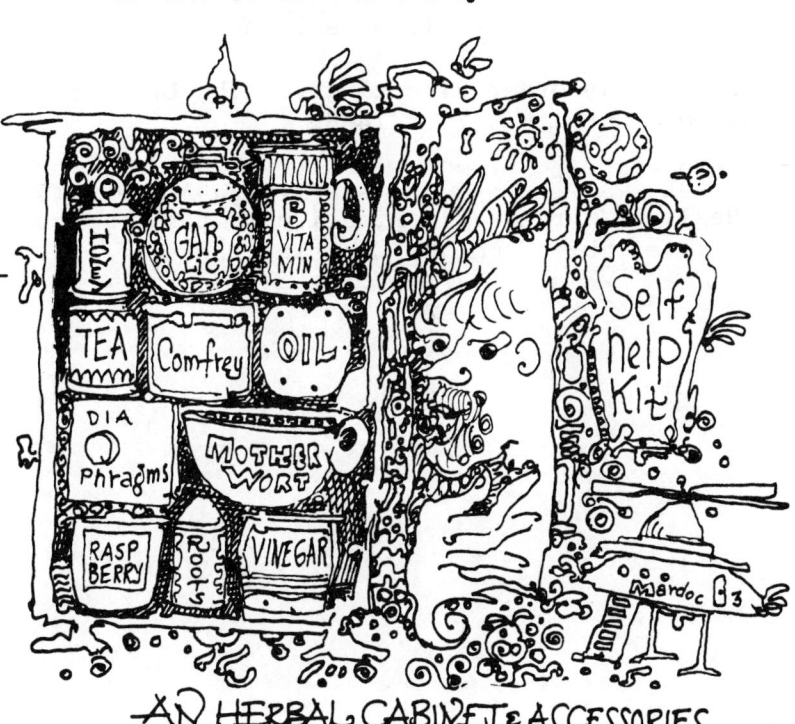

AN HERBAL CABINET & ACCESSORIES

ALSO BY JOY GARDNER:

<u>A Difficult Decision, A Compassionate Book About Abortion</u>, $6.95.

<u>Healing Yourself in Pregnancy</u> (coming in 1987 from The Crossing Press)

Write to Healing Yourself Distribution Company, Box 952, Vashon, Wash. 98070 to order these. In Canada, order from Healing Yourself Distribution Company, 811 Victoria Street, Nelson, British Columbia.

Or you may order directly from The Crossing Press, P.O. Box 640, Trumansburg, New York 14886.

A catalog of books and products which Joy recommends is available from Healing Yourself Distribution Company. A catalog of books and cards is available from The Crossing Press.

YOUR OWN REMEDIES

YOUR OWN REMEDIES

YOUR OWN REMEDIES

INDEX

Aches, 4
Anemia, during pregnancy, 47
Antibiotic alternatives, 11
Ascorbic acid, 2
Aspirin alternatives, 5
Asthma, 14-15

Babies
    diet, 17
    problems, 16-17
Bacterial sore throats, 11
Bacterial vaginal
    infections, 37
Baldness, 25
Basal body temperature, 39
Belly-aches, 8
Birth control, 39-41
Bladder infections, 35
Boils, 26
Bones, children's, 17
Books to read, 64
Bruises, 26
Bumps, 4
Burns, 27

Calcium, 58
Cervicitis, 37
Chest congestion, 6
Childbirth, 42-52
Children's problems, 16-17
Cobalamin, B_{12}, 55
Colds, 2-3
Colic, 16
Congestion, 6
Constipation, 18
Cosmic fertility cycles, 41
Coughs, 7
Cradle cap, 16
Cramps, 38
Cystitis, 35

Dandruff, 25
Diaper rash, 16
Diaphragm, 41
Diarrhea, 19
Dietary guidelines, 32-33
Diuretics, 47
Dizziness, 9

Eczema, 27

Fasting, 19
Fats and oils, 44
Fertility cycles, 41
Fevers, 12
Foreskin, 17

Gas, 8
Genital itching, 29
Gingivitis, 13

Hair, 25
Headaches, 5
    during pregnancy, 47

Hemophilus, 37
Hemorrhoids, 20
    during pregnancy, 48
Hepatitis, 22-24
Herpes, 30-31
Hits, 4
Home deliveries, 49-50

Infants, 16-17
Insomnia, 34
Intestinal flu, 8
Iron, 57
    baby's, 51
    during pregnancy, 44
IUD cramps, 38

Laxatives, 18
Leg cramps, 48
Liniment, 4
Lower bowel tonic, 18
Lung massage, 15
Lung tea, 15

Magnesium, 58
Menstrual cramps, 38
Morning sickness, 47
Migraine headaches, 5

Nasal congestion, 6
Natural fertility cycles, 11
Nausea, 9
    during pregnancy, 47
Nervous tension, 34
Niacin, B_3, 55
Non-specific vaginitis, 37
Nursing babies, 52
Nutrition, 32-33

Parasites, skin, 4
Perineum, 51
Piles, 20
Pinworms, 21
Post-natal care, 51
Pregnancy, 42-52
Preventative medicine
    for asthma, 14
    for colds, 2-3
Protein, during pregnancy, 44
Providing nourishment, 32-33
Psoriasis, 27
Pubic area itching, 29
Pubic hair itching, 29
Pulse, 14
Pyorrhea, 13
Pyridoxine, B_6, 55

Restlessness, 34
Rhythm method, 39
Riboflavin, B_2, 54

Scabies, 4
Sinus congestion,
Sinus headaches, 6
Skin, baby's, 51

Soreness, 4
Sore throats, 10-11
Sprains, 4
Staph infections, 28
Stomach-ache, 8
Stomach flu, 8
Stomach upset, after meals, 8
Strains, 4
Stress, 34
Swellings, 4
    during pregnancy, 47

Tapeworms, 21
Teeth, 13
    children's, 17
    during pregnancy, 47
Teething, 17
Tension, 34
Thiamine, B_1, 54
Throat, sore, 10-11
Toothache, 13
Toxemia, 47
Tranquilizers, 34
Trenchmouth, 13
Trichomonas, 37

Umbilical cord, 51
Urination, frequent
    during pregnancy, 47
Urinary tract infections, 35

Vaginal infections, 36-37
Varicose veins, 48
Viral sore throats, 10
Vitamin A, 53
    during pregnancy, 44
Vitamin B, 54-55
    during pregnancy, 45
Vitamin C, 56, 2
    during pregnancy, 45
Vitamin D, 56
    during pregnancy, 45
Vitamin E, 57
    during pregnancy, 45
Vitamin K, during pregnancy, 45
Vomiting, 8-9

Worms, 21

Yeast infections, 36

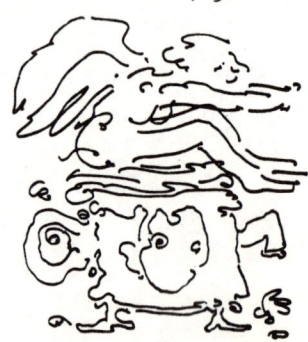